Get in touch with yourself through

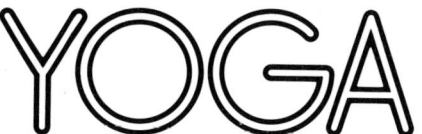

Get in touch with yourself through

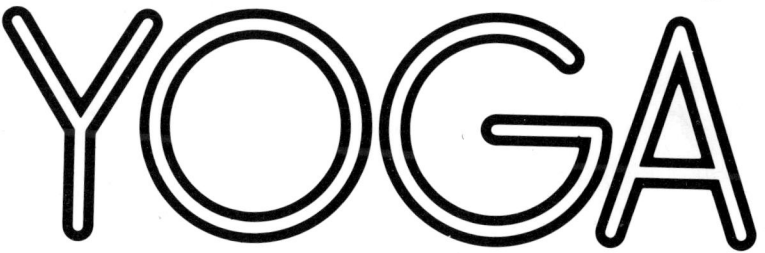

A Modern Programme for Total Health and Well-Being

By Tillie Mia

William Luscombe Publisher Ltd
In Association with Mitchell Beazley Ltd

Dedication

*With love to my family, to Harriette for getting me in,
to Cecile for helping me out, and to my ever-present,
indispensable Dutch-English dictionary.*

Photographs by Reginald Wickham

Original American edition published by
Prentice-Hall, Inc. New Jersey.
First British edition published by
William Luscombe Publisher Ltd.
The Mitchell Beazley Group,
Artists House,
14–15, Manette Street,
London, WC1V 5LB,
1974

ISBN 0 86002 005 3

Contents

6

Introduction

Never in my wildest dreams did I expect to write a book—
especially in English, which is not my native language. So
what am I doing behind a typewriter, writing about Yoga of
all things? After all, I am not a guru. Nor do I sleep on nails
or try to hold my breath for half an hour. If I did, I would
have been a corpse long before now—although not a bad-
looking one I must add in all modesty, for never in my thirty-
nine years have I felt or looked better. And staying attractive
certainly isn't easy, not while living in this neurotic and
pressured world of today, and even worse, in the heart of mad,
frantic, and polluted New York.

But what has all this to do with Yoga? Isn't Yoga a
mysterious philosophy that suggests one stand on his head or
contemplate his navel? There is indeed the very beautiful
Yoga philosophy in which man forever searches into the
purpose of his existence, seeking to train the body and the
mind to the highest degree of perfection.

This book, however, will be concerned with the perfection
of the body, so we will merely concentrate on Hatha Yoga,
which envelopes the physical development of our being,
always combined with the Pranayama, or breath control, and
Savasana, the deep relaxation of body and mind. To be a true
Yoga scholar requires a complete devotion and dedication,
which in our Western world is extremely hard, if not virtually
impossible to achieve. But reading this book might make you
so enthusiastic that before you know it, you're on the next
plane to India. In the meantime, while you are still here, I
will try to take part of the beauty of Yoga, its power and
benefits, and apply it to our hectic way of life to help you make

7

it as tranquil and healthy as possible and to help you feel revitalized and younger.

How did I become interested in Yoga and what has it done for me? Let me go back a few years. I was born and raised in Holland. At the end of World War II, I was a very skinny girl and my mother immediately made up for all the hungry years by having me eat everything that was fattening, absolutely convinced that if you're not fat you must be sick. For a while I completely enjoyed this abundance of food. I was perfectly happy and not for a moment regretted the fact that I was chubby. Nor did it seem to bother a handsome American student. We fell in love at first sight and got married two years later in Amsterdam. After my husband finished medical school, we went to the United States, me very fat and pregnant. You see, Dutch doctors did not make mothers-to-be miserable by putting them on diets. Therefore, I ate merrily during the day, and during the night a bit less merrily only because I was sleepy. It was sheer heaven. I gained forty-five pounds and gave birth to a beautiful baby girl. I did not give much thought to the fact that when I left the hospital I still had to wear maternity clothes! Twelve months later I was back in the hospital to give birth to this incredibly ugly baby, who is today my very handsome son. This time I had only gained forty pounds thanks to the strict supervision of my doctor, who gasped in total disbelief every time I stepped onto the scale. He had absolutely no understanding of the fact that I had just discovered halavah in my new country and simply could not stop eating it. Guess what I wore when I left the hospital?

Since my husband was then a resident physician, we had very little money and we were living in hibernation in the Berkshire Mountains of Massachusetts. So there was little else to do but to make another baby. Forty pounds later, a tiny, skinny girl was born. After this was all over, I was a respectable 175-pound heavy lady. My husband claims I was beautiful, but, of course, love is blind. Taking care of three babies helped melt twenty-five pounds off me within a year, and I decided to live graciously with the other 150, considering it my fate. Because I stem from a family of marvellously jolly though rather portly women, I accepted this plumpness as an inherited characteristic.

8

Before I became involved in Yoga I had joined several exercise classes. The problem was that not only did I begin to look like Tarzan, but, because I was absolutely exhausted, I could barely drag myself home after each class. And, of course, the moment I entered the house, I was bombarded with questions such as, 'Why can't we ever have spaghetti for breakfast?' or 'How come you never take us to an X-rated movie?' Naturally, I was supposed to stand there like a pillar of strength, while all I wanted to do was to go to bed. But all this came to a premature ending. While I was doing some marvellous contortion on the rings, my back went out, and that finished gymnastics for me.

Then I met a woman who introduced me to Yoga and became my teacher. I loved it from the very start. My body began to feel more limber and youthful. Inspired by this power over my body and the feeling of well-being, I also began to eat more sensibly and gradually lose weight. My figure became firm and tight, and needless to say, it needed a lot of tightening. The deep Yoga breathing induced such a feeling of good health that smoking cigarettes seemed an interference. So for me the practice of Yoga breathing, and quite a lot of willpower, made me give up smoking. Today I am healthier, slimmer, and more energetic than ever before.

Besides being a teacher of Yoga, I am now also a mother of teenagers. In both cases I'm standing on my head at times— as a mother, either out of despair or in side-splitting laughter, since this certainly is a varied and rocky stage with all its difficult as well as utterly delightful moments.

Naturally I have been eager to create an interest in Yoga for teenagers. The main reason is that I strongly feel that there is not enough emphasis on physical education in their lives, and that many schools do not have adequate facilities for it. Granted, the young people learn to play football, basketball, and what other games have you, which is great, but it is not sufficient for the total development of their fast-growing bodies. Physically this is a very awkward time for them, as it is difficult to coordinate those suddenly long arms and legs. They feel rather insecure and clumsy about their bodies which makes it hard for them to move gracefully and with confidence. Therefore I recommend Yoga as much for young people as for adults.

I clearly remember the first teenage class I taught. There in front of me were these seven wonderful, long-haired creatures, sitting most comfortably and relaxed in the Full Lotus position (their teacher as well, though not as comfortably) when I noticed the slight movement of a jaw. I gently brought to the attention of the class that it was not wise to chew gum during a Yoga lesson, and seven hands simultaneously went to seven mouths to take out the gum, which was then stuck on to the most unbelievable places, and from there on did we proceed to do our first Yoga posture. I very soon learned that although their bodies were very limber, their muscle control and coordination was very poor indeed.

Accompanied by the expected moaning and groaning, we had a most delightful lesson as I began to teach them better control and greater awareness of their bodies, strongly emphasizing the importance of good posture.

I hope they will remember some of it throughout the years. 'Find us young, keep us so' I read somewhere in Bartlett's *Familiar Quotations*.

Unlike most other ways of exercising, Hatha Yoga is done in slow motion. (The movements are called postures, rather than exercises.) One moves slowly into a position, holds this for several seconds, and comes out of it equally slowly. It is the gentle stretching and contracting of the muscles that makes them stronger and more elastic. By gradually increasing the length of time for holding a posture, one builds up the endurance, strength, and flexibility of the body.

Because of the slow motion of Yoga, our bodies will tell us exactly what our limits are, and consequently, help us to avoid pulled ligaments, strained tendons, and painful backaches. It is for this reason that Yoga can be practised by young and old—by anyone reaching for the ultimate of his body's potential. In Yoga one aims for a limber and healthy body— and with consistent practice we can keep in excellent shape and slow down the ageing process. I realize that is quite a statement to make, but it is like the farmer who every night carried his newborn calf into the barn and continued to do so until it was full grown. When people admired his great strength, he answered, 'I never felt the calf get heavier since I carried him every day.'

As opposed to many active sports that can cause strain on

the body and therefore fatigue, Yoga works out the body completely and reduces all tension. However, I very much urge you to participate in sports. Not only is it a great physical and emotional outlet, but it seems to be one of the very few things left in this world that unites people of all classes, races, or colours—even if only for a short moment. And Yoga can help you increase your proficiency in the sports you like. There are, for instance, excellent leg exercises which might turn out to be of great benefit to you on that icy ski slope. Or, if you play tennis, perhaps you will not be out of breath so soon, since the Yoga postures and breathing improve the blood circulation dramatically, and give you more endurance and clearer concentration.

Yoga values and places tremendous importance on strengthening and working out every part of the spine. The Yogi believes that a strong and limber spine makes our movements graceful and is the secret for a strong body and youthful appearance. After learning the Yoga postures, you will discover that you'll be able to move more spontaneously and naturally and will feel better all day long. All of us are aware of how important it is to keep our bodies in good shape, not only for aesthetic reasons, but especially for our health. And since life expectancy is getting longer, how much more fun it is to keep fit and limber long enough to enjoy it. And of all the marvellous benefits Yoga can give you, one of the most important and little known is that it controls the accumulation of toxic acids, therefore helping to keep the arteries elastic. 'All right,' I hear you say, 'so I'll have elastic arteries,' but if I tell you that this will play a big role in preventing the hardening of the arteries, you won't know how to turn these pages fast enough so you can start exercising like mad.

Of course, you shouldn't expect miracles. But Yoga has been good for me, and I believe it will be good for you also.

Chapter One

The discipline of Yoga frees the mind from distracting thoughts and teaches it to concentrate on the moment that is now.

Yoga: When, Where, and How

The moment has almost arrived when you can practise your first Yoga posture. But don't do so right after getting up from the dinner table as it might turn out to be rather uncomfortable. You must always give yourself enough time to digest your meals well.

In fact, it is preferable that Yoga be practised on an empty stomach, so the best time to choose is either in the morning or before you go to bed. In the morning, because Yoga stimulates the blood circulation, and the increased intake of oxygen that goes along with deep breathing will refresh the brain and help you start the day bright and alert. And since Yoga postures limber your body from head to toe and improve your posture dramatically, you will go to work erect, full of energy, and feeling great. Now, if you don't find a parking ticket on your car, the dustbin knocked over, or any other such disturbing realities, you might have the beginning of a perfect day.

If it is more convenient for you to practise at night, do so before you go to bed. You will find that Yoga helps you to relax and unwind. Slowly it works out all the tension that has gathered in areas such as the neck, shoulders, and back. Your breathing will become deeper and more regular, and will prepare you for a lovely night of deep, restful sleep. Do I seem to be contradicting myself—one moment speaking about how Yoga will revitalize you and the next about how it can put you to sleep? I'm not. There are particular exercises that will regulate the heartbeat and have a sleep-inducing effect on you and these I will specify in a special chapter later in this book.

I did write previously that Yoga can be practised at any age. In fact I consider it almost a necessity for people over forty, since I have seen in my teaching how rapidly ageing and inactivity can limit the body's movements. Even though Yoga can limber the body again to a great extent, it takes time and consistent work. If, however, one practises Yoga regularly, I am definitely convinced that the body will stay supple, flexible, and youthful for many years. And what can I say? Since it is the only body you have, you might as well take good care of it.

To get back to where I started, Yoga can be practised at any age. In case you have had a recent operation, illness, or serious back trouble, consult your physician before indulging in Yoga. Most likely the decision will be in favour of Yoga— particularly for back problems—provided it is done in moderation, without any force or strain.

Where shall you do your Yoga? Theoretically, you should always do the postures in a quiet, well-ventilated area, on either a carpeted floor or a hard surface that is covered by a blanket or a large towel. But we can do much better than that. How about Yoga in your garden on a glorious spring morning, surrounded by crocuses and daffodils and the loveliness of eager, budding, tender, young greenery, accompanied by the jubilant songs of birds. I also highly recommend Yoga on the beach if you are so lucky as to have it all to yourself (you might gather quite an audience if you do it on a crowded beach). For instance, a few years ago, some friends, my husband, and I chartered a sailboat in the Caribbean and sailed the Virgin Islands for ten days. In the late afternoons we would drop anchor close to one of the many beautiful little islands. With the sun going down in all its magnificence, never did life seem more lovely and tranquil. I would swim to the beach, and then, facing the sun and the ocean, almost touching the edge of the water, I would deeply breathe in the clean, pure air and start my Yoga. One day I did not notice that a large sailing yacht had dropped its anchor—I did not notice partly because I was concentrating intensely on my Yoga and partly because I am rather nearsighted. And until they were very close, I did not see the man in the rowboat dropping off a case of ice cold beer 'with the compliments of the captain—he enjoyed watching you.' Now it so happened that we had run out of ice and were for several days drinking lukewarm cokes, orange juice, and what other horrors have you. So I think 'rewarding' can be added to the many virtues that Yoga has claimed for itself.

What to wear. Obviously a bathing suit when on the beach. At any other time preferably leotards. Something magical seems to happen the moment one gets into leotards. One can imagine oneself a great dancer, or absolutely flip over that sexy image that is smiling back in the mirror, or decide that very moment to go on a crash diet. There is a wide selection of the most exciting colourful leotards now on the market. Anyway, never wear anything tight, confining, or uncomfortable.

Naturally, once your friends find out that you are practising Yoga you can be sure they will ask for a demonstration. In fact, you might even be rather eager to volunteer. After all, some Yoga postures are very beautiful, others are intricate, and some are very amusing. Quite a temptation to show off. But don't. First of all, it might turn out to be rather uncomfortable in tight clothes and especially with peanuts and a martini in your stomach. But it can also be reckless, since at such a time you do not have the concentration and balance required for the Yoga postures. So save it for the next morning, when your mind is bright and clear.

Last, but not least . . . laugh! I believe so much in the therapeutic power, restoring quality, and disarming effect laughter has on all people, no matter where they live or what language they speak. Laughter teaches us not to take life too seriously, that every one of us at times feels miserable and alone, that most of us have the same fears, doubts, and hopes. Sometimes laughter prevents us from crying, and ultimately it gives us the knowledge that tomorrow will be better.

So laugh when you can't reach your toes with straight knees, or can't keep your legs up in the air. Don't ever feel ridiculous or that it is hopeless. It will all happen gradually.

Work slowly but consistently on your Yoga postures. It is a matter of stretching the muscles, limbering the spine, and building endurance.

Try to practise every day. With a daily minimum of twenty minutes and a little bit of effort, you will soon experience exciting results.

Chapter Two

The slow but consistent practice of Yoga can lift us to the highest level of performance.

Five Fundamental Yoga Postures

There are five basic Yoga postures that by the very nature of their total involvement of each part of the body structure create a most beneficial result. It is for this reason that I prefer to describe these postures now, for in themselves, the combination of these five postures will give the body a profound, overall workout. At a later time you may wish to use these five fundamental postures when you only have time for a brief Yoga session.

It is important, however, not to rush into the practice of these postures. If you are going to try them now work at them very slowly, and *do not strain* to do any part of a posture that you find difficult. At the end of the book there is a developmental programme through which one gradually prepares the body for the increasingly more difficult postures. Remember that it is only through consistency, patience, and perseverance that one will reach the ultimate goal of control and perfection.

Salutation to the Sun

It is good to start the Yoga postures, or the day for that matter, with this beautiful exercise, so lyrically called Salutation to the Sun. This combination of postures will limber the entire body—especially the spine—and prepare you well for the Yoga postures that follow. Learn to breathe correctly with each posture and you will find this a most refreshing and invigorating way to stay fit, agile, and alert.

Practice Technique
Stand erect, palms and feet together (Fig. 1A).

16

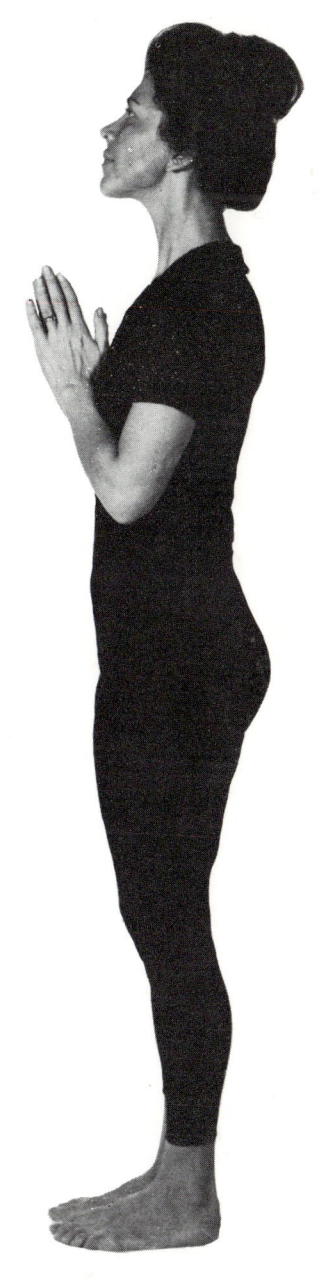

1A

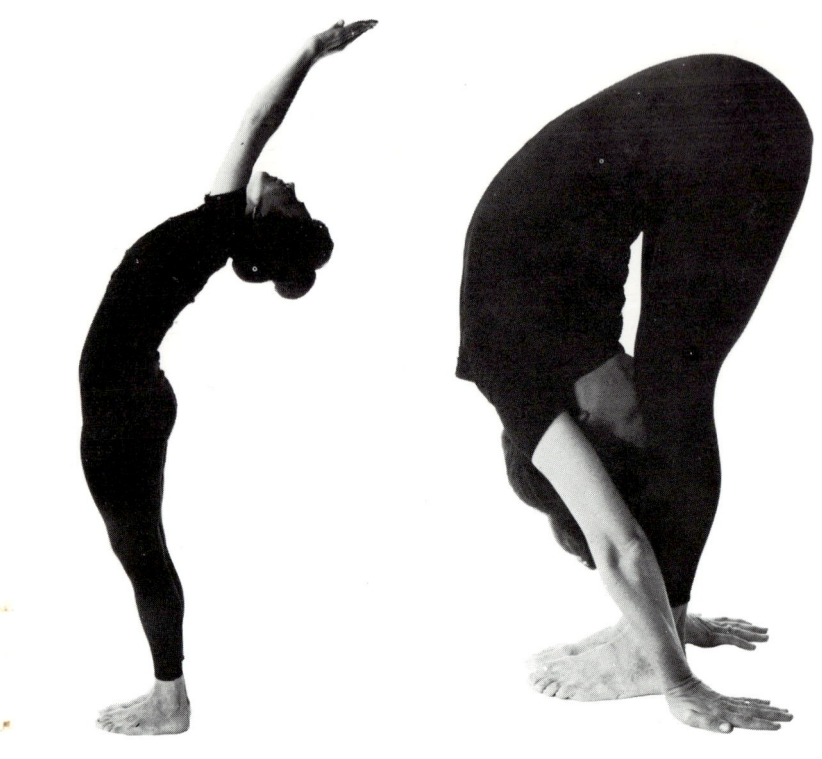

1 B   1 C

Inhale deeply, raise your arms over your head, and bend backward (Fig. 1 B).

Exhale and bend forward, keeping your knees straight at all times. After enough practice you may be able to touch your hands to the floor and your forehead to your knees (Fig. 1 C).

Inhale deeply, stretch your left leg behind you, look up, and press your right thigh against your abdomen (Fig. 1 D).

Exhale and move your right leg behind you as well, supporting your body with your arms (Fig. 1 E).

Inhale and slowly lower your body. Touch your chin to the floor and raise your buttocks slightly (Fig. 1 F).

Hold your breath and bend the upper part of your body as far back as possible (Fig. 1 G).

Exhale and raise your body high, keeping your toes on the floor and your head between your arms (Fig. 1 H).

18

Inhale and lower your trunk, while bringing your left leg forward and pressing your thigh against your abdomen (Fig. 1I). Look up.

Exhale and raise your trunk and buttocks as high as possible, while bringing your right leg forward to meet your left (Fig. 1J).

Inhale while straightening up. Stretch your hands way over the head and lean backward (Fig. 1K).

Exhale and come back to the first position (Fig. 1L).

Repeat at a slow and even cadence.

The Lotus Position

This position is most essential, for it is here that the spine is at its most erect, which is absolutely terrific for a good posture. The particular advantage of it is that one can hold this position for any length of time and sit in it while reading, talking, watching TV, or writing a book for that matter. The Lotus is also the basis of several other Yoga postures that will be described in later chapters.

There are three Lotus positions: The Easy Pose (Fig. 2A) in which one simply sits in a cross-legged position; the Half Lotus (Fig. 2B) in which one places one foot on the opposite thigh; and the Full Lotus (Fig. 2C), in which each foot is placed on the opposite thigh. I must confess that the Full Lotus is very difficult for most people including myself, and I could hardly wait to get the picture over with! So do sit at length only in the position that is most comfortable for you and practise the more difficult ones only for a short period at a time.

The Swan

I consider the Swan a most beneficial posture for the entire body. It works out the chin, neck, arms, chest, spine, abdomen, pelvis, legs, feet, and even feels wonderful. What more can one ask for?

Practice Technique

Sit in your comfortable Lotus position. Clasp your hands together behind your back, tighten your abdomen, and raise your arms as high as possible, keeping your chin way up (Fig. 3). Inhale deeply, hold this posture for a minimum of ten seconds, exhale, and relax.

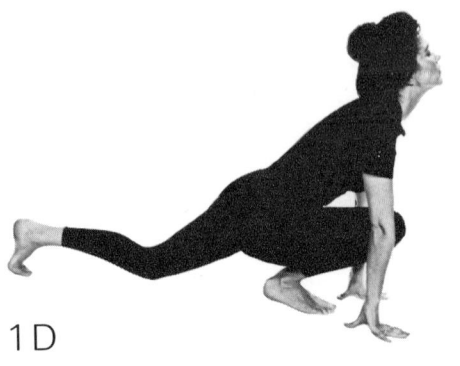

1D

1F

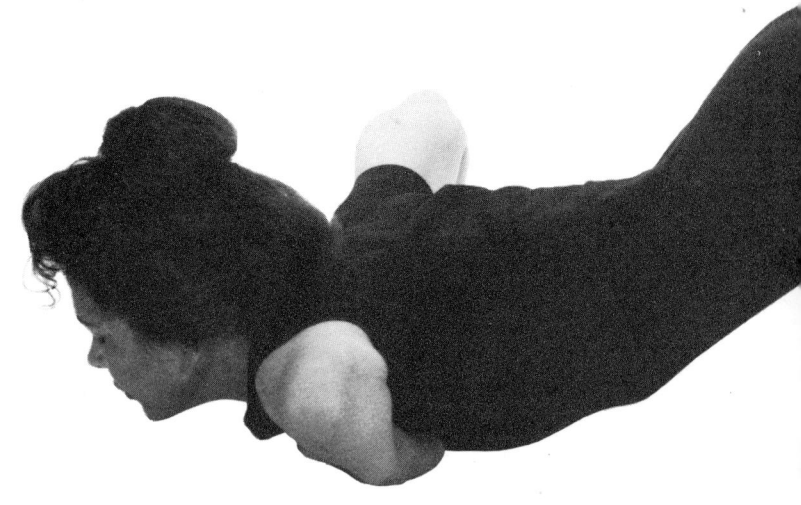

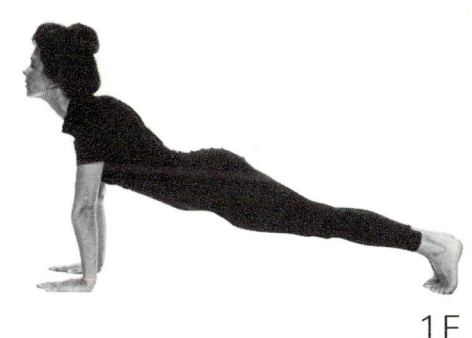

1E

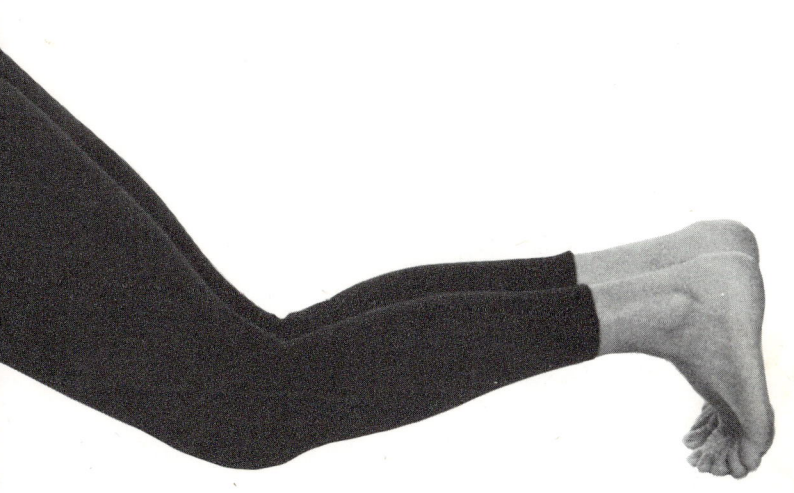

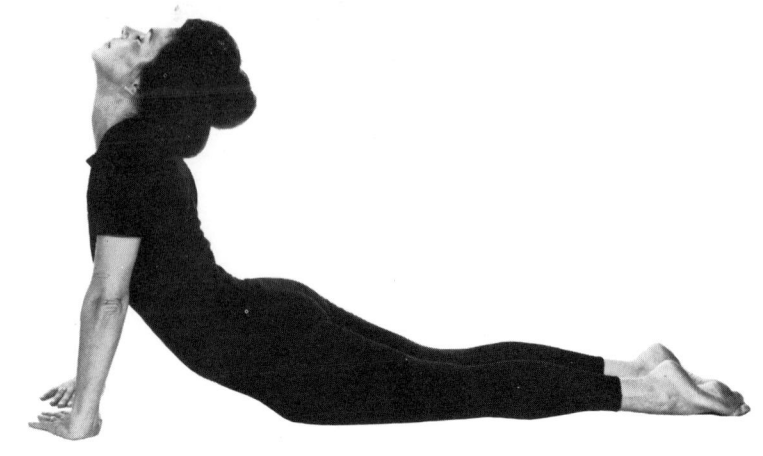

1G

1H

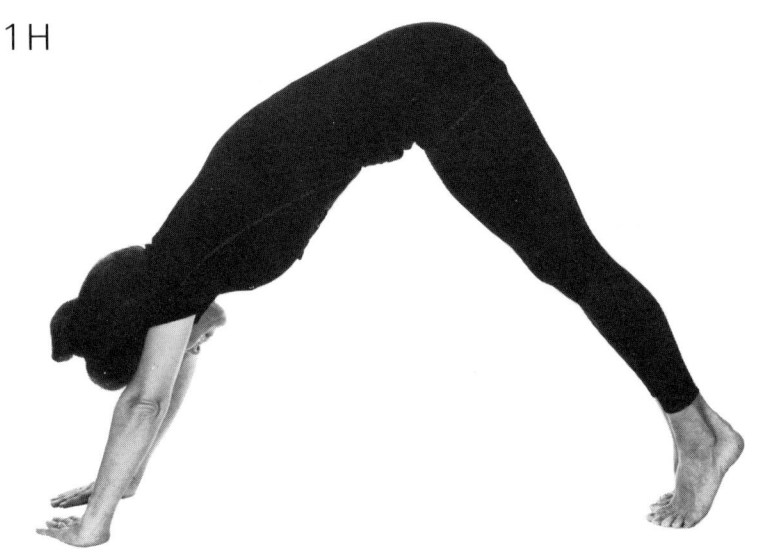

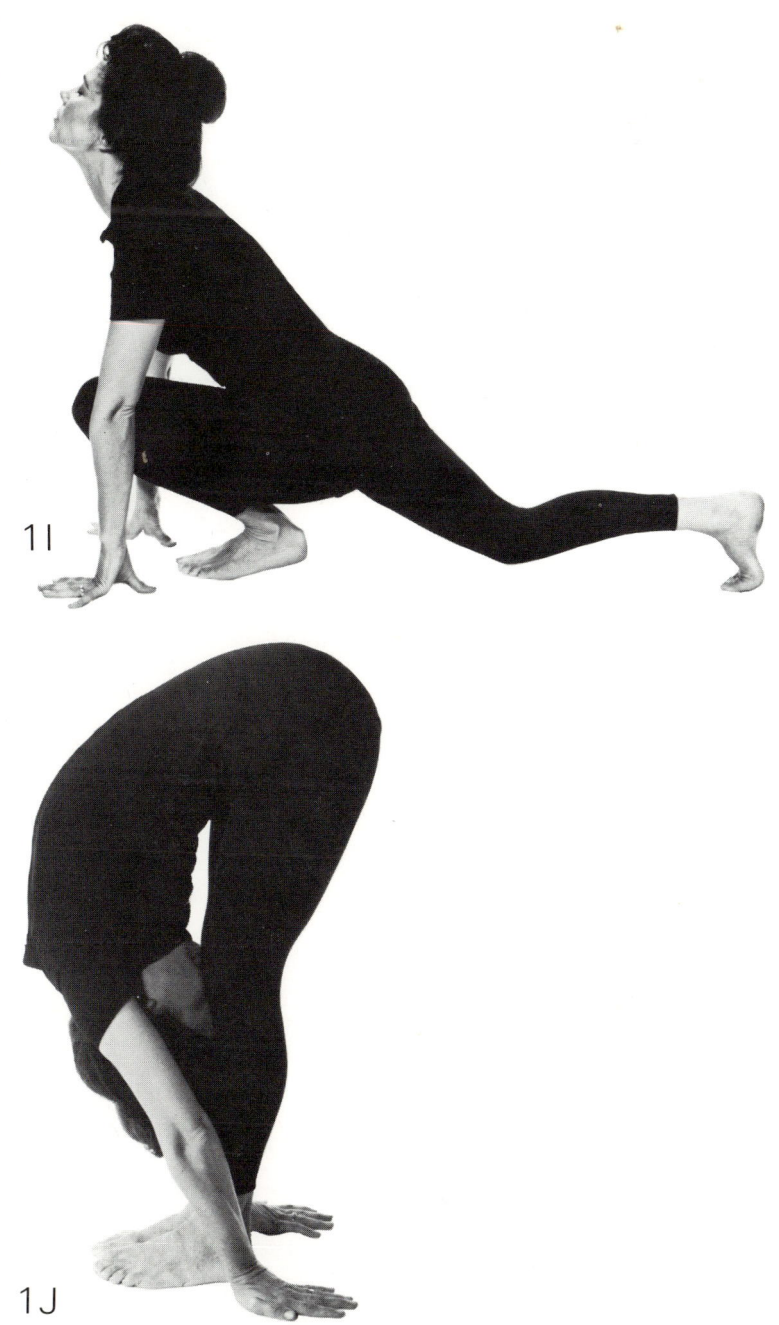

1I

1J

23

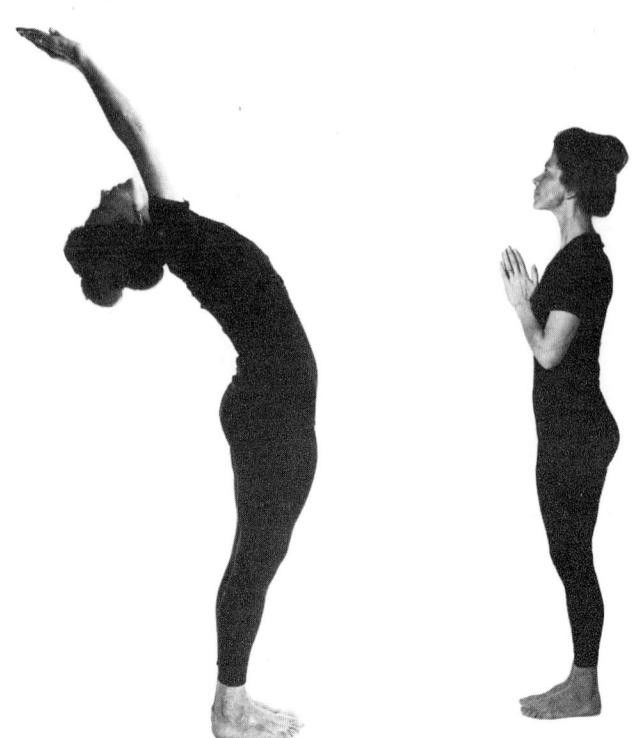

1K   1L

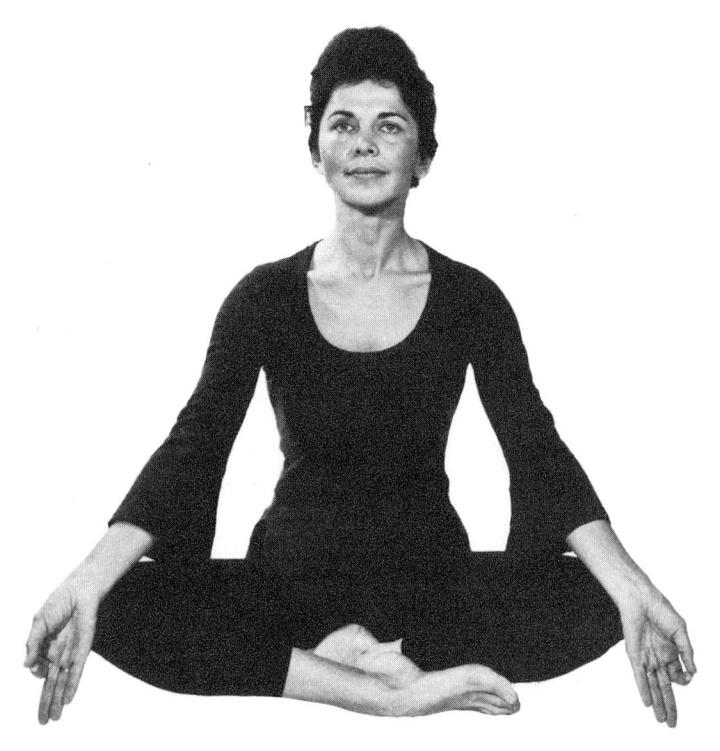

2A

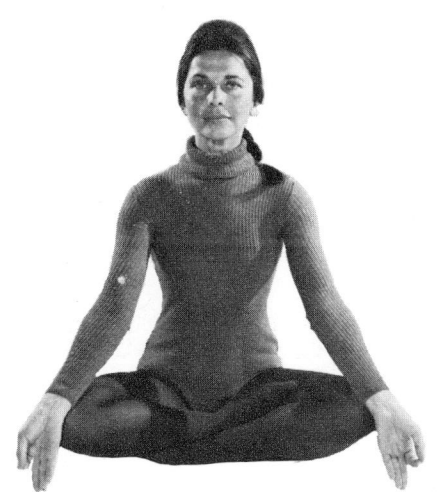

2B

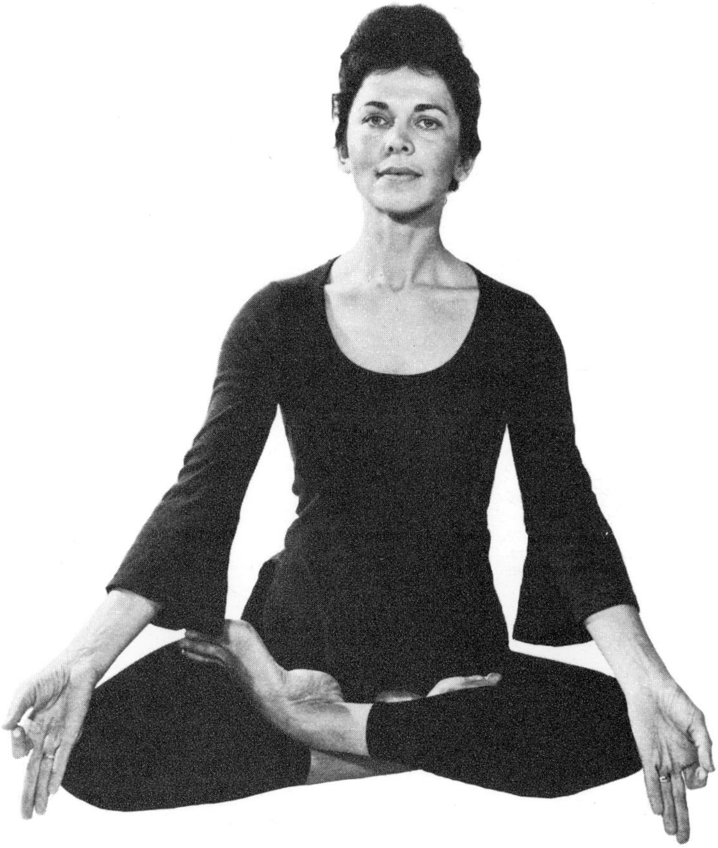

2C

The Shoulderstand

If one has only very little time to practise Yoga, never leave
out the Shoulderstand. For few Yoga postures match its
profound influence on the entire body. Not only will the
Shoulderstand strengthen the spine and stimulate the blood
circulation, but it is an excellent help in preventing and
reducing varicose veins. It also works out tension that has
gathered in the neck and shoulders and helps to regulate
menstrual disorder.

The Shoulderstand is especially known for the effect it has
on the thyroid gland, as the chin lock stimulates its functioning. The Shoulderstand therefore becomes a most important
posture in the attempt to lose weight, providing it is practised
daily for a minimum of three minutes.

3

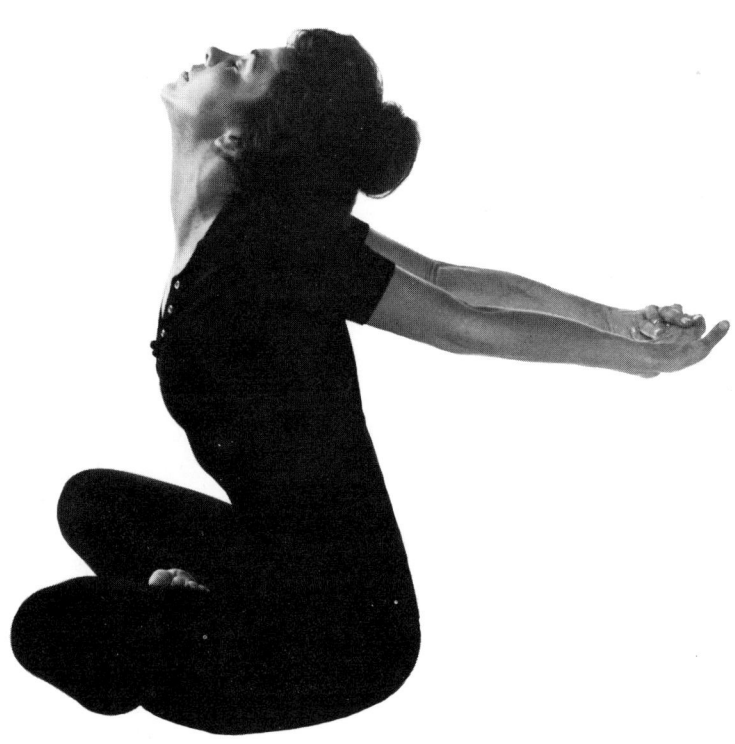

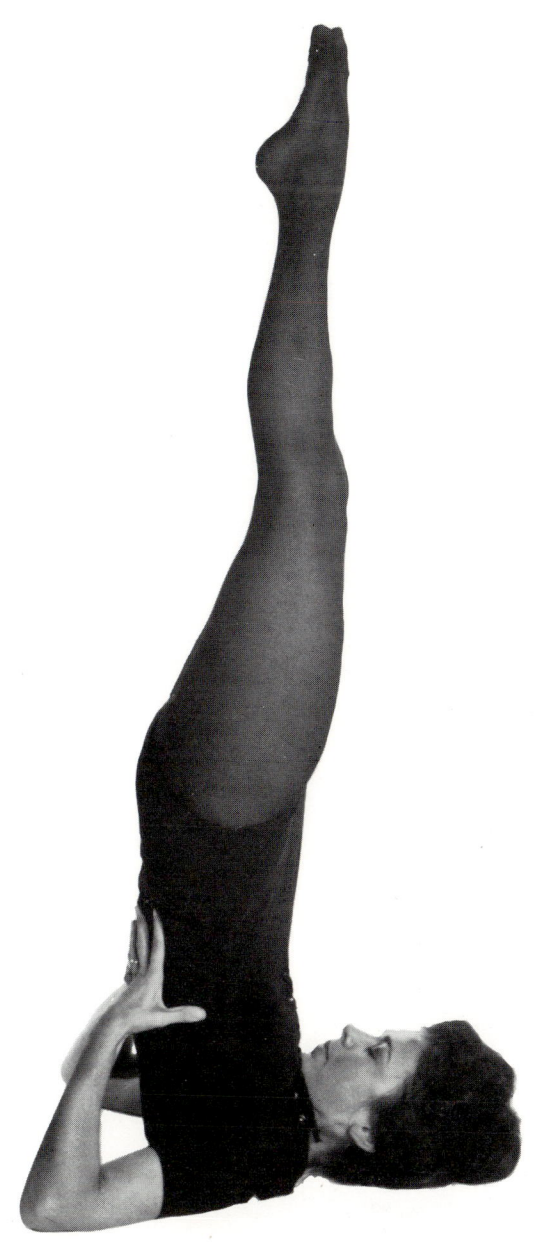

4A

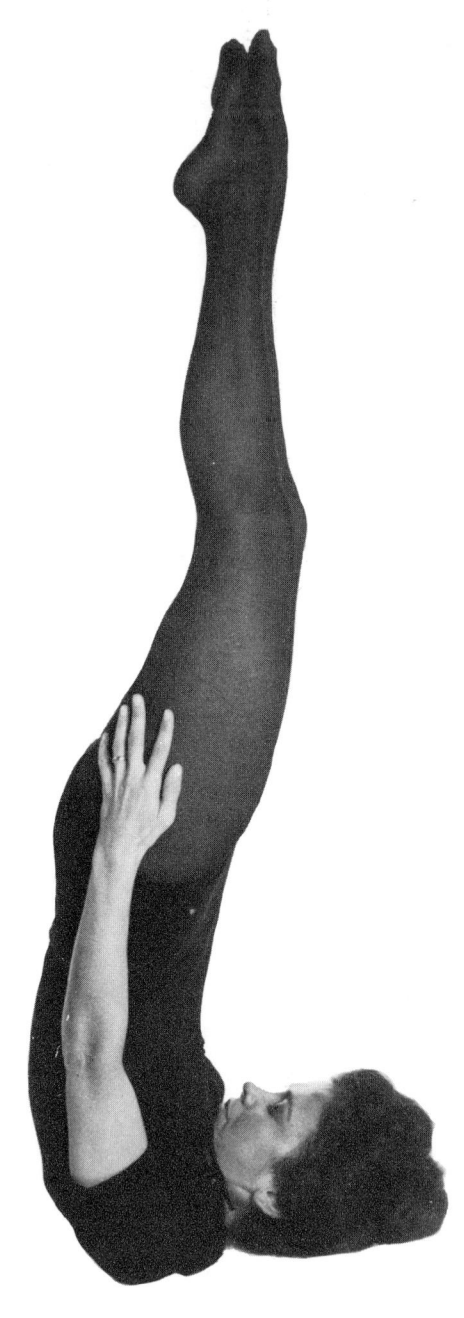

4B

Practice Technique

Lie flat on your back, hands alongside your body. Slowly raise your legs, hips, and trunk, swinging them beyond the vertical position before straightening the body out. Support your back with both hands (Fig. 4A). Continue to breathe deeply and hold this posture for thirty seconds, increasing the time up to three minutes over a period of a month.

To come out of this position, arch your head back slightly, bring your knees to your forehead, place your arms in front of you on the floor with the palms down. Then, balancing yourself with your hands, slowly and gracefully lower your trunk to the ground. When your trunk is down, keep your legs up at a ninety-degree angle and take twenty seconds to lower them slowly to the floor, a fantastic abdominal exercise in itself. Breathe deeply, close your eyes, and relax until your heartbeat has become regular.

The Advanced Shoulderstand and the Bridge Pose

After you master the Shoulderstand with ease and comfort, slowly remove your hands from the support of your back and place them vertically alongside the body (Fig. 4B), concentrating deeply on maintaining your balance.

From this position you now will lower yourself into the Bridge Pose. Start by supporting your back firmly again with your hands. Now bend your knees and slowly lower one leg at the time until your toes touch the floor. When the toes of both feet are on the floor, hold this posture for fifteen seconds (Fig. 4C).

4C

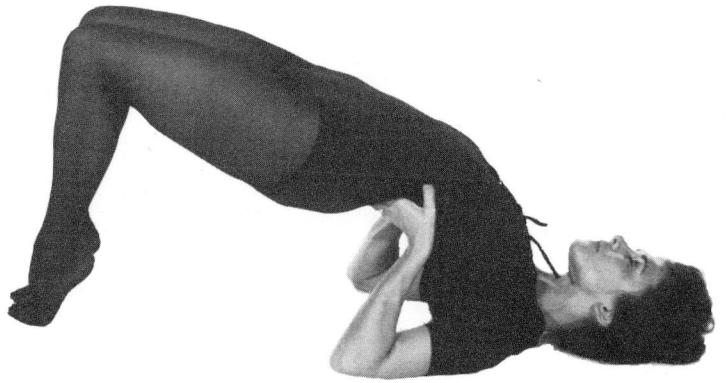

The Headstand

Even though you don't *have* to stand on your head to do Yoga or to receive its over-all benefits, I will not deprive those who desire to defy the laws of gravity the opportunity to learn the Headstand!

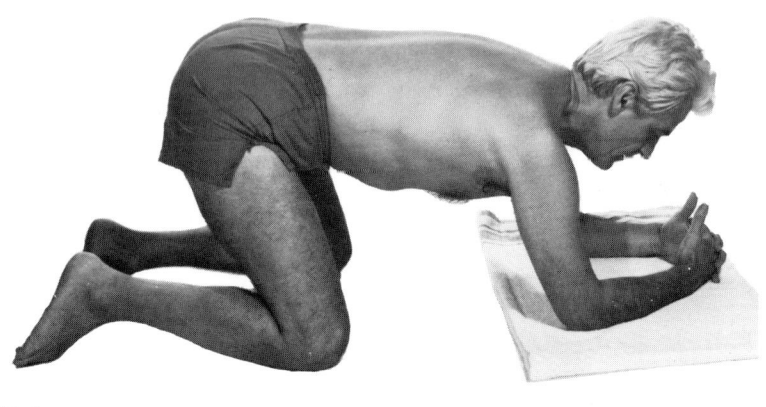

5A

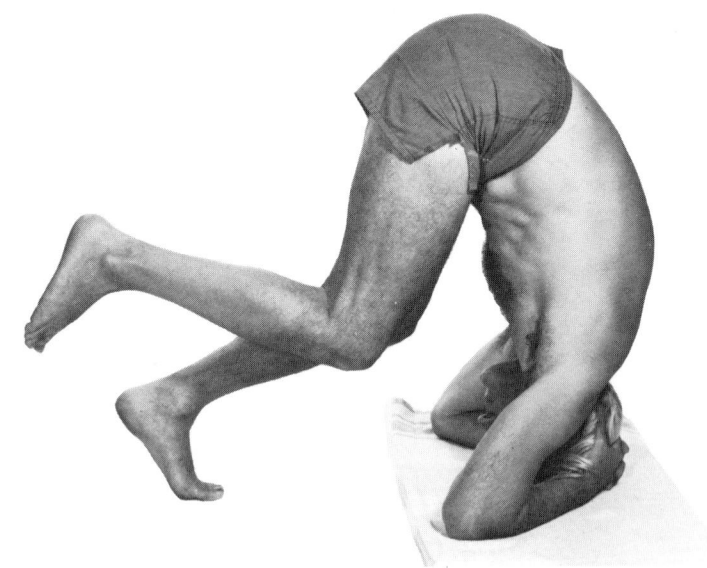

5B

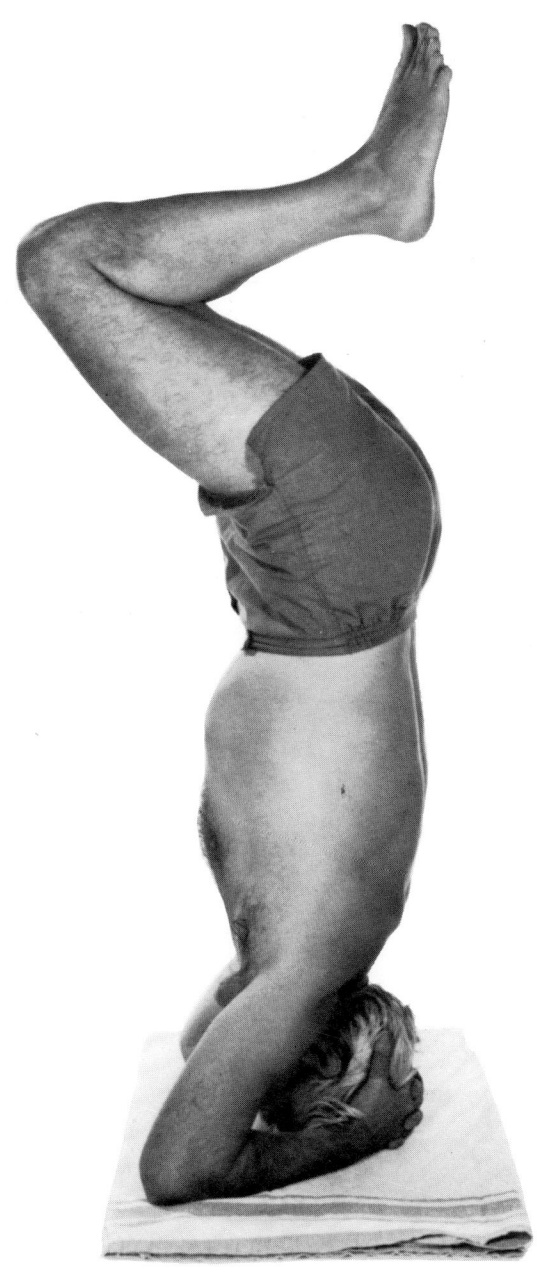

5C

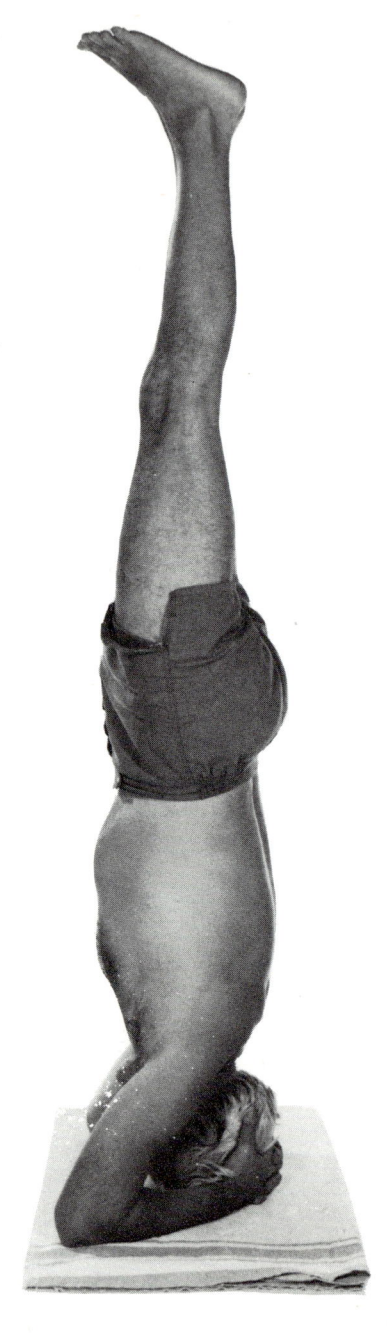

5D

The effect and benefits of the Headstand are similar to those of the Shoulderstand, with the addition that it leads a rich supply of blood to the brain, therefore increasing its thinking ability and sharpening the power of concentration.

However, before you become too daring, remember that *each stage* of the Headstand should be practised for several weeks. By all means, *do not rush into it*. It is best to practise in a corner, so that you have two walls to give you support, until you are completely secure in your mastery of the art of standing on your head.

Practice Technique

Place a folded towel on the floor and kneel in front of it. Put your forearms on the floor, angling them slightly toward each other, and intertwine your fingers (Fig. 5A).

Cradle the back of your head firmly into your clasped hands, stand up on your toes and walk inward in order to bring your knees close to your chest.

This movement will raise the trunk automatically into an upright position (Fig. 5B).

You will feel that by gently lifting your toes off the ground, the momentum will bring your trunk into a perfect vertical position (Fig. 5C). Do not try to straighten up your legs yet. Concentrate intensely on maintaining your balance, dividing the weight of your body between your head and forearms. After you are able to hold this posture steady for two minutes, proceed by slowly straightening your legs into an upright position (Fig. 5D). At first remain for fifteen seconds in each position shown in Figures 5C and 5D. Gradually increase the duration of the Headstand itself to five minutes.

To come down, slowly bend your knees and place your feet softly on the floor. Remain in a kneeling position with your head resting on the floor, for at least one minute, in order to harmonize the blood circulation.

Chapter Three

Yoga follows the wisdom of the tree that bends with the force of the wind, patiently resting as it creates the energy to restore itself.

Development of the Spine

The central axis of our body is the spinal column. Together with its ligaments, vertebrae, and associated muscles, it supports the entire body through its anti-gravitational function. Because of its flexibility it also becomes the very basis of agility and youthful and graceful movements.

However, in our daily lives we often neglect the possibility of moving the spine in a way it was designed to be used. The result is a stiff, rigid, and very often weak backbone which does little else but support our weight.

Many people suffer from weak and painful backs. I know a number of extremely active and athletic people who suffer from severe back discomfort. Some of them play quite a game of tennis, others are skilful skiers or excel at some other physical sport.

The reason they have backaches is that most sports involve the use of one particular set of flexor, extensor, or rotator muscles of the spine while the other sets which are not developed become relatively nonfunctional. This creates disequilibrium in the development of the spine and easily leads to sprains, tears, and muscular damage.

Yoga, on the contrary, equally develops each of these groups, resulting in a more flexible and stronger spinal column, which is less liable to injury.

One thing I can pride myself on is a tremendously strong back which enables me to carry and move rather heavy objects. It always seems to surprise gallant men to see this deceivingly helpless-looking woman carrying such heavy boxes or grocery bags. When they offer their assistance, they practically collapse right in front of me with an expression of great wonder in their eyes, and I am sure, regretting ever being so chivalrous! But all the proud and mighty come to a fall, and one day while working in the garden I caught a case of lumbago and by the end of the day I could barely walk straight. The next morning when I crawled out of bed, my legs went right out from under me. This got me mad, especially since the next day I would have to teach Yoga to a class of beginners, and it does sound sort of funny to be told your Yoga teacher had to cancel because her back went out.

So I sat down and slowly started to work on the Yoga postures, stopping the moment I felt pain. It must have been quite a sight, for I felt a hundred years old. But gradually I was able to straighten up, became more limber, and felt much better throughout the rest of the day. The next morning I still had difficulties getting out of bed, but decided to grin and bear it and not call off the class.

However, I first went through the whole routine of a beginner's lesson to work out my back and to find what my weak point was. I was all right until I got to the Shoulder-stand. I expected to crack right on the spot. The question was, how could I possibly teach a Yoga class without a Shoulderstand—after all, the least a Yoga teacher can do is to introduce herself standing on her head. I tried once more and found that if I pulled my knees up high, I could wrap my arms around them and bend down my forehead as if to touch the knees, thus rolling myself into a ball in order to roll back and forth several times (a great back exercise in itself by the way). While going back the fourth time the momentum brought my legs up into the air without any pain and I was able to perform a sublime Shoulderstand.

Anyway, my pupils had a complete Yoga lesson given by an erect, confident (only I knew better) and—if I remember correctly—even a smiling teacher (I told you I'd grin and bear it)!

This incident proves to me that the slow and gentle Yoga postures can be most soothing and effective for back discomfort.

Anatomically, the spine can be divided into four parts.
1. Cervical or neck area.
2. Thoracic or upper part of the back.

3. Lumbar or lower part of the back.
4. Pelvic and sacral area.

You will find a specific set of Yoga postures on the following pages which will help develop each particular area in concave, convex, lateral, or rotational directions.

Remember once more, never force, strain, or go to the extent that a posture becomes painful. I want you to feel good not only after, but during exercising. You will find that each day you will reach, bend, and stretch a little further. Work on it with patience, perseverance, and . . . pleasure. And by the way, many of the postures always have to b(repeated on either the left or the right side, depending on what side you started out. I don't want you to grow crooked now!

The Cobra
This particular posture symbolizes the amazing flexibility of

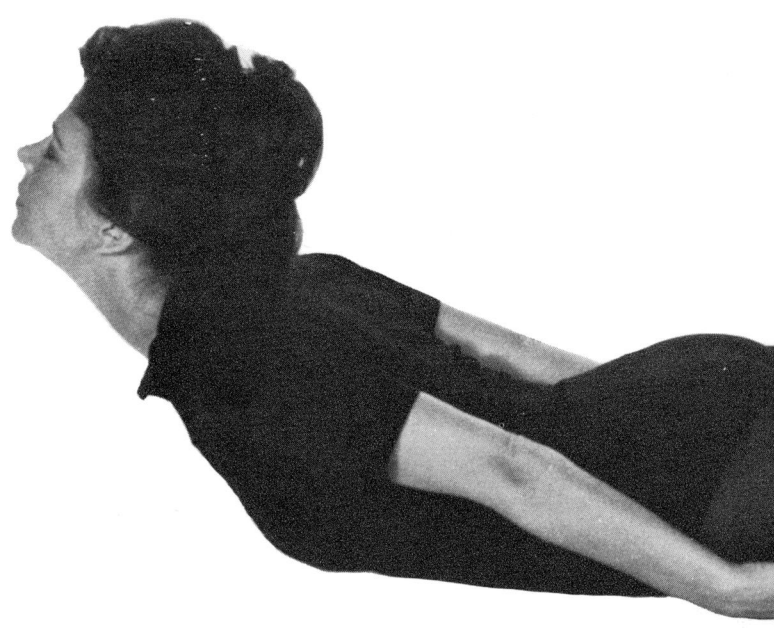

6A

a cobra's spine, encouraging you to strengthen and limber your own. Needless to say, one must not expect to obtain the mobility of a snake.

Instead, this posture creates a marvellous sleep-inducing effect. So if you cannot fall asleep, stop counting sheep and perform the Cobra three times, followed by the Alternate Nostril Breathing (which you will learn later), and you will sleep like a baby.

Practice Technique
Lie on your stomach, forehead on the floor, arms alongside your body. Your feet should remain close together.

Slowly raise your forehead off the floor, followed at an extremely slow pace by your chin, neck, shoulders, and chest (Fig. 6A). Bring your arms forward until your hands are in front of you palms down, with the fingers pointing toward

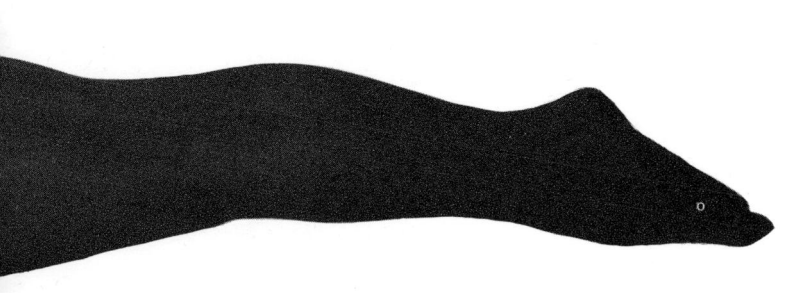

each other. Now, equally slowly, in one flowing motion, use your arms to help raise the upper part of your body as far as you possibly can, bending your head way backward as well (Fig. 6B).

Hold this position for five seconds, then return to starting position in the exact but reversed manner. When your fore-

6B

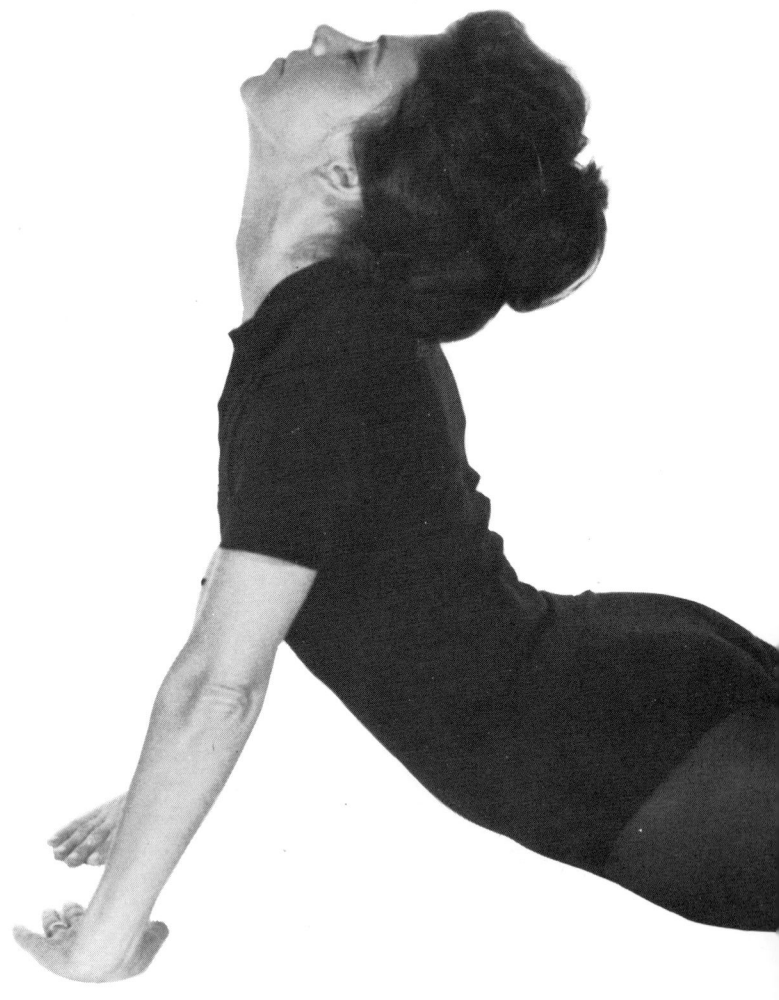

head reaches the floor, close your eyes and relax until your heartbeat has become regular.

For the first week, increase the holding time to fifteen seconds. In succeeding weeks, gradually increase to fifty seconds.

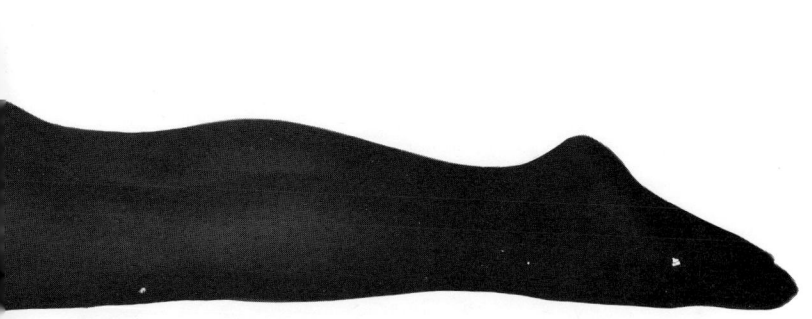

The Plow

At first glance, the different stages of the Plow might seem virtually impossible, but I assure you that they are quite a bit easier than you expect them to be. The Plow is a good example of the gradual but steadily progressive effect Yoga has on the body. You will find that through continuous practice you will become increasingly limber and comfortable in the three postures of the Plow. Start practising with the first stage. Never force or strain your body, but hold this pose for as long as you comfortably can. After you feel at ease, proceed to the second stage, and again maintain the posture for as long as you wish.

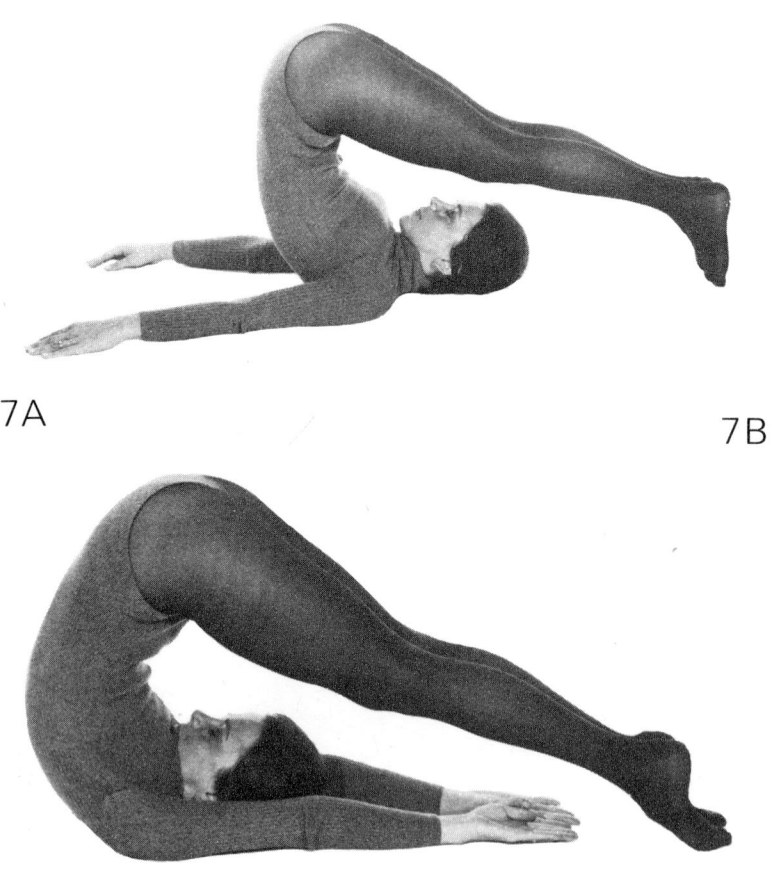

7A

7B

Eventually conclude this lovely exercise by going into the third stage. You may find this a most pleasant position to be in, and rest assured that the Plow is one of the most beneficial and effective Yoga postures for strengthening, limbering, and development of each and every area of the spine.

Practice Technique
First Stage
Lie flat on your back, keep your arms alongside your body, and slowly start to raise your legs, with your feet together and knees straight.

Bring your legs up and over your head and try to bring them down behind your head as far as possible, ideally having your toes touch the floor (Fig. 7A).

Try to relax your neck, close your eyes, and breathe regularly. At first hold this position for ten seconds.
Second Stage
While in the first stage, try to 'walk' your legs several inches away from your head and bring your arms above your head, placing them flat on the floor, palms up (Fig. 7B). Once again, relax your neck, continue to breathe regularly, and start off by holding this position for ten seconds.

7C

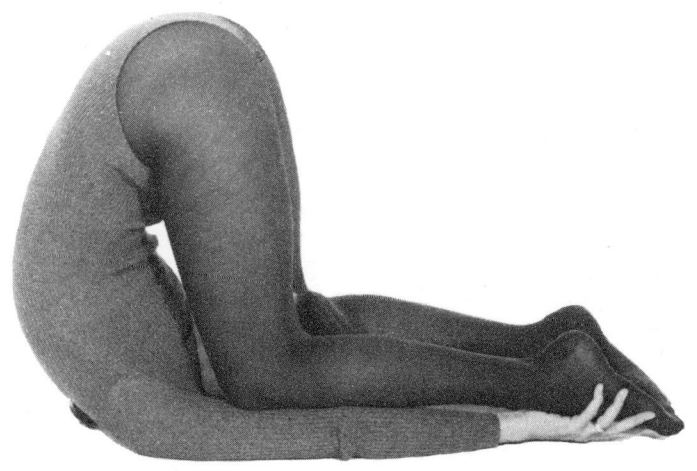

Third Stage

From the second stage we now bring the knees forward next to the ears (Fig. 7C). Hold for ten seconds.

In order to come down, arch your neck backward, bring your hands to the front of you and close together on the floor, palms down. Slowly lower your trunk to the floor in one flowing movement. When your legs are at a 90-degree angle from the floor straighten out your knees and take twenty seconds to bring your legs down to the floor. Relax, breathe

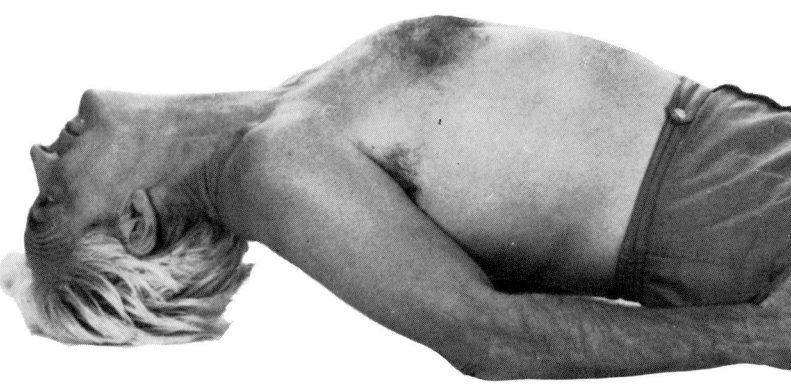

8A

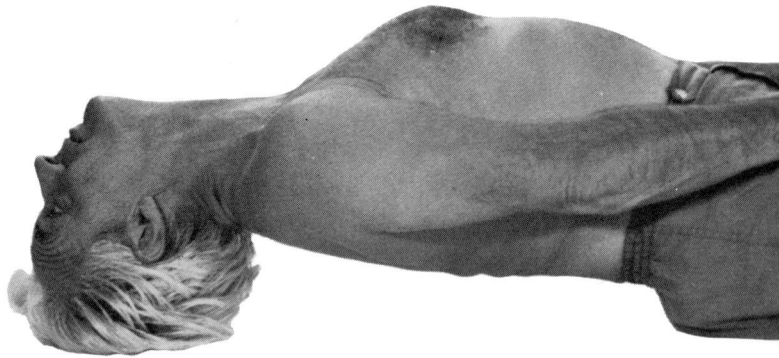

8B

deeply, and wait until your heartbeat has regulated itself.

The Fish

Why this posture is called the Fish I cannot tell you, but the fact remains that it is a most effective way to remove tension and stiffness in the neck, shoulders, and the cervical region of the spine. It is recommended that you practise this posture after you have been in the Shoulderstand in order to counteract the convex bend of the neck.

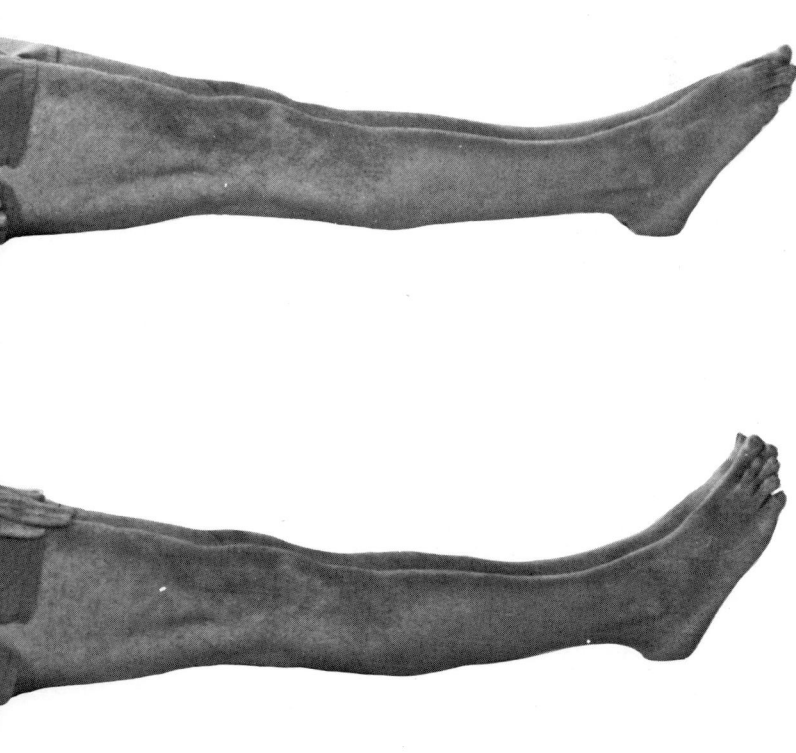

Practice Technique
Lie flat on your back with your arms close to your body. Place your weight on your elbows, lift your trunk upward and bend your head completely backward, until it touches the floor, creating an arch between your head and buttocks (Fig. 8A). Hold for ten seconds. After practising this posture for several weeks, add a final step: Lift your elbows slowly off the floor, place your hands on your thighs, and hold (Fig. 8B).

In order to come down, support your body by leaning on your elbows again, slowly raise your head, bring your body down, and relax the spine. Breathe deeply.

The Half Spinal Twist
I do admit this to be a rather intricate posture that could create the impression that one is trying to compete with a pretzel. However, its rotating movement exercises and limbers the entire spine, stimulating the deep as well as superficial muscles of the back at the same time.

Always keep in mind that although the back carries the entire body with ease, it remains a most delicate instrument, and at no time should one force, strain, or jerk in a posture. As a rule, nature is kind enough to give the body a warning by creating discomfort in case of excessive strain. Be wise enough to listen!

Practice Technique
Sit on the floor with both legs stretched out in front of you. Fold your left leg inward, placing the sole of the foot close to your groin. Bend your right knee, take your ankle in both hands, carry your foot over the folded left leg, and place your right foot to the outside of your left thigh with the sole flat on the floor.

Turn the left shoulder to the right in order *to touch the left* foot with the left hand. Swing your right arm around the back and take hold of your waist on the left side, and turn your head to the extreme right. Hold this posture for five seconds and slowly come out of it, by returning your head to the centre, relaxing the arms, unfolding your legs and straightening them out in front of you.

Repeat the posture on the opposite side.

Gradually increase holding time for this posture to twenty-five seconds. After you are comfortable enough to remain in this posture for as long as twenty-five seconds, advance to the Full Spinal Twist.

The Full Spinal Twist

Go through the same leg movements you use for the Half Spinal Twist. Now bring your left shoulder forward and your

9A

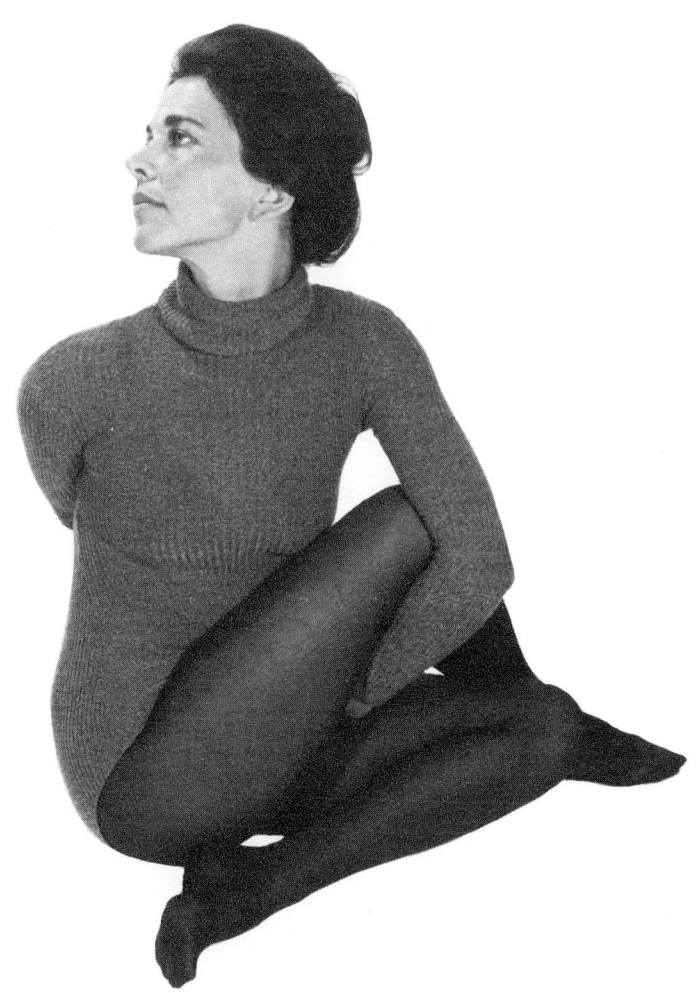

left arm over your right knee. Guide and insert your left hand and arm under and through the back of your right knee (Fig. 9A).

Swing your right arm around the back of your waist and try to have your hands meet each other in an attempt to eventually clasp them together (Fig. 9B). Turn your head to the extreme right and hold the posture for five seconds.

Come out of this posture by returning your head to the centre, unclasping your hands, relaxing your arms, unfolding your legs and stretching them out in front of you. Relax and repeat the posture on the opposite side.

With continued practice, gradually extend the time for holding this posture to twenty seconds.

9B

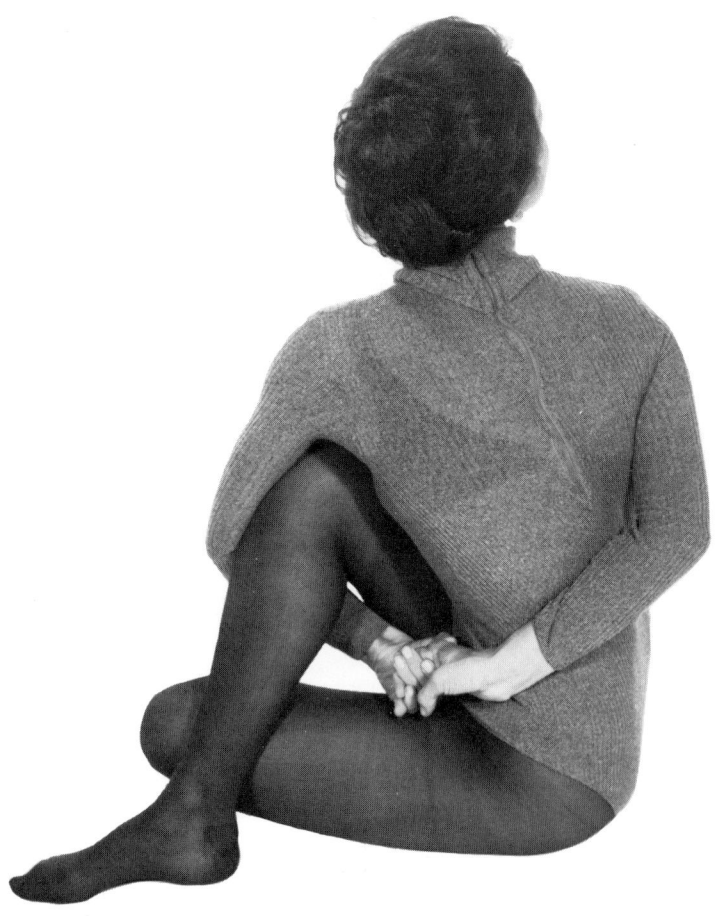

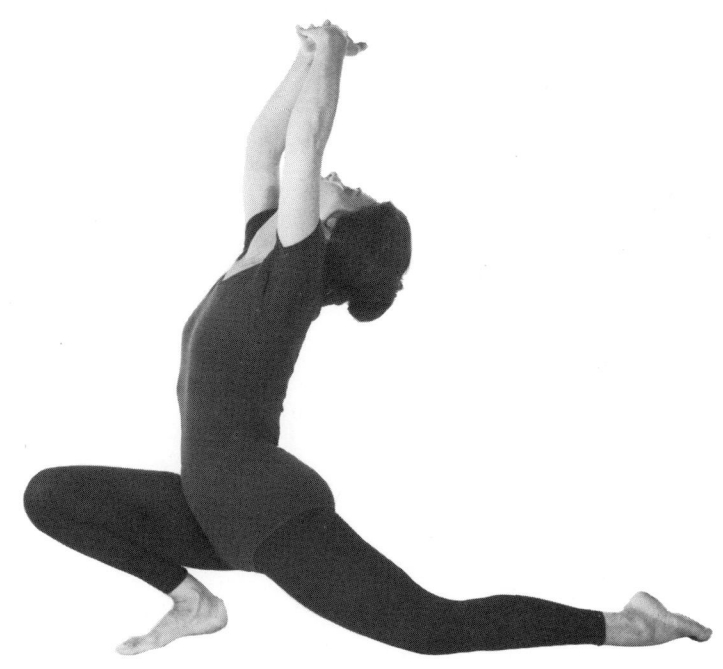

10A

The Monkey Posture

This posture gives the entire spine a beautiful concave and lateral stretch, and it also works out stiffness in the legs.

Practice Technique
Kneel down on your left knee and place your right leg, with the foot flat on the floor, in front of you.

Shift your weight on to your right leg, simultaneously raising your arms over your head. Intertwine your fingers. Look up and slowly bend backward as far as you are able to, and hold for ten seconds (Fig. 10A). Slowly turn your head to the left, looking back toward your left foot, while bringing your arms down sideways and toward your back. Then grasp your right wrist with your left hand (Fig. 10B). Once again, hold this pose for ten seconds, and gradually, with practice, increase the time to forty seconds.

Alternate by kneeling on the right knee and repeat.

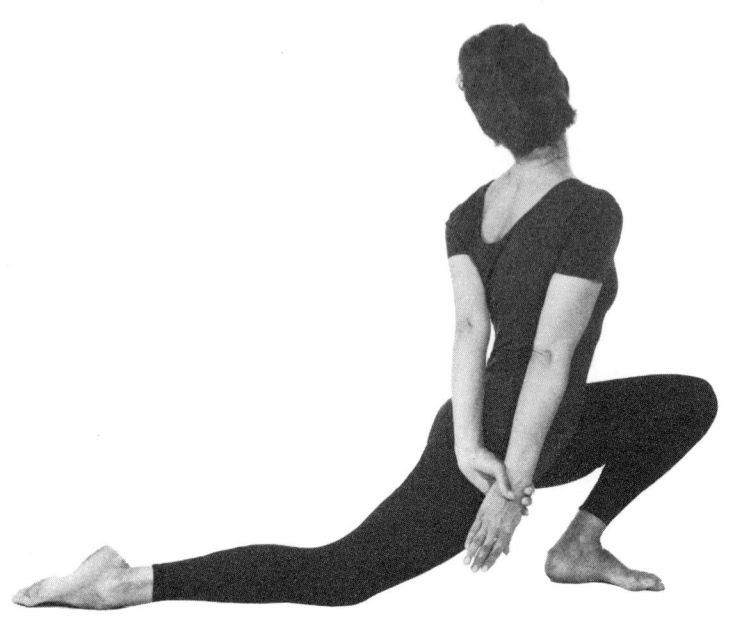

10B

The Cat

A very gentle posture that massages the spine beautifully.

Practice Technique

Rest on all fours. Bend your head away down between your arms, slowly forming a high, round back (Fig. 11A). Tighten your abdomen and inhale deeply.

Hold for five seconds.

Bring your head way up high so that the back forms a hollow (Fig. 11B), exhale, and hold the posture for five seconds. Repeat the entire posture four more times.

48

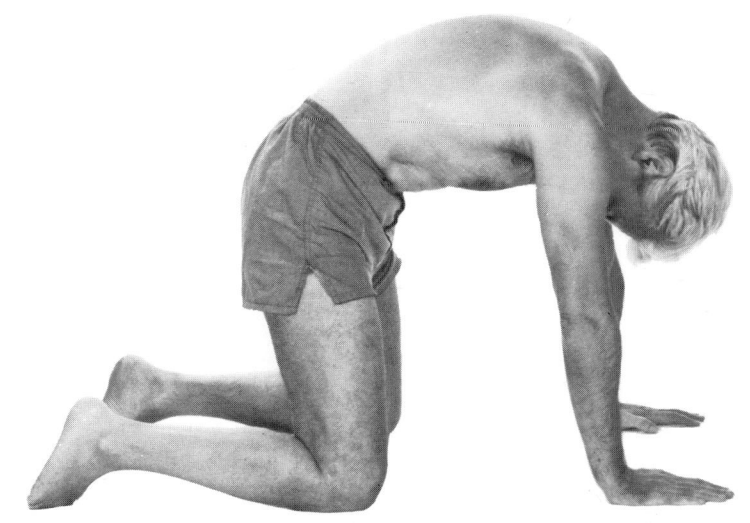

11A

11B

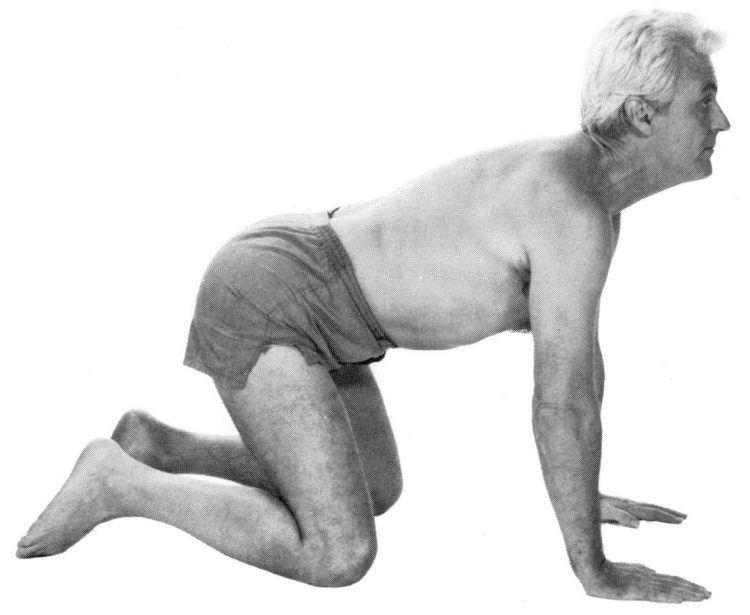

The Head-To-Knee Pose

This posture works out the lower part of the back extremely well and its enormous stretch creates a lengthening effect on the entire spine, reminding you of the fact that as the body ages, the spine compresses and therefore gradually becomes

12A

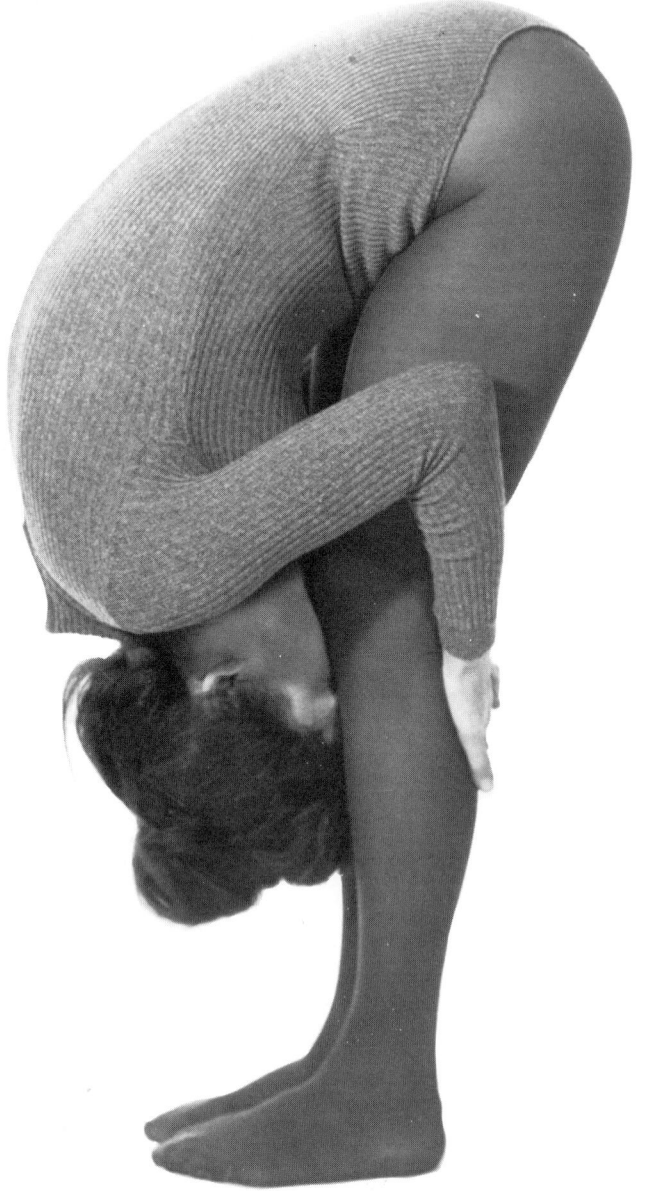

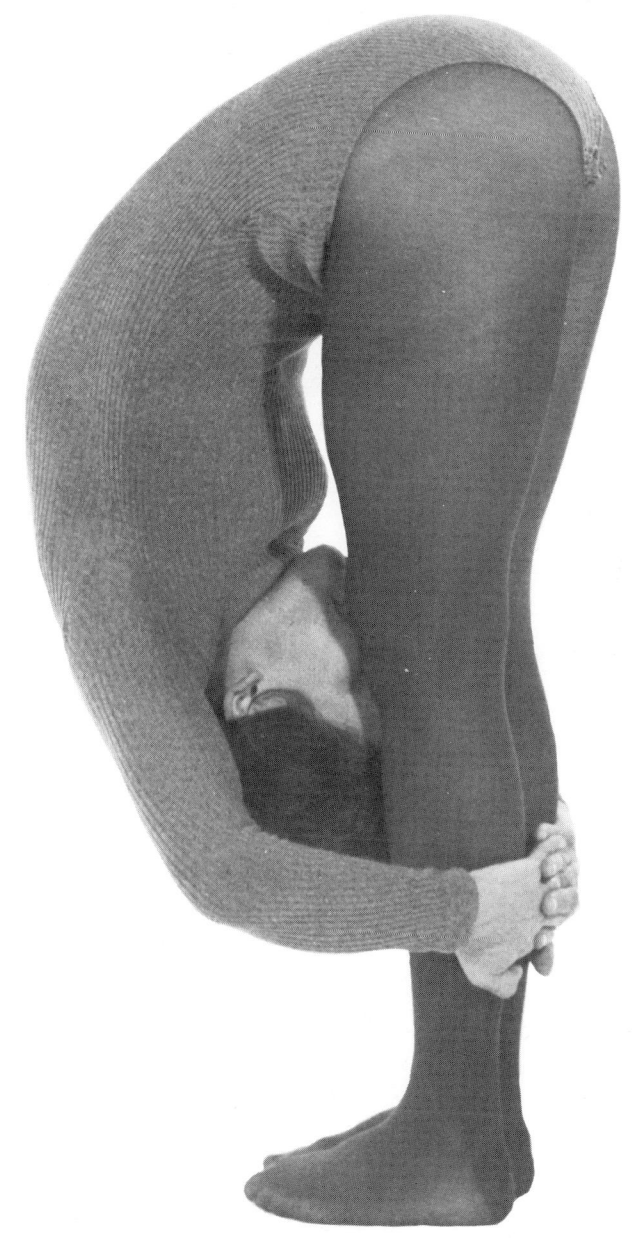

12B

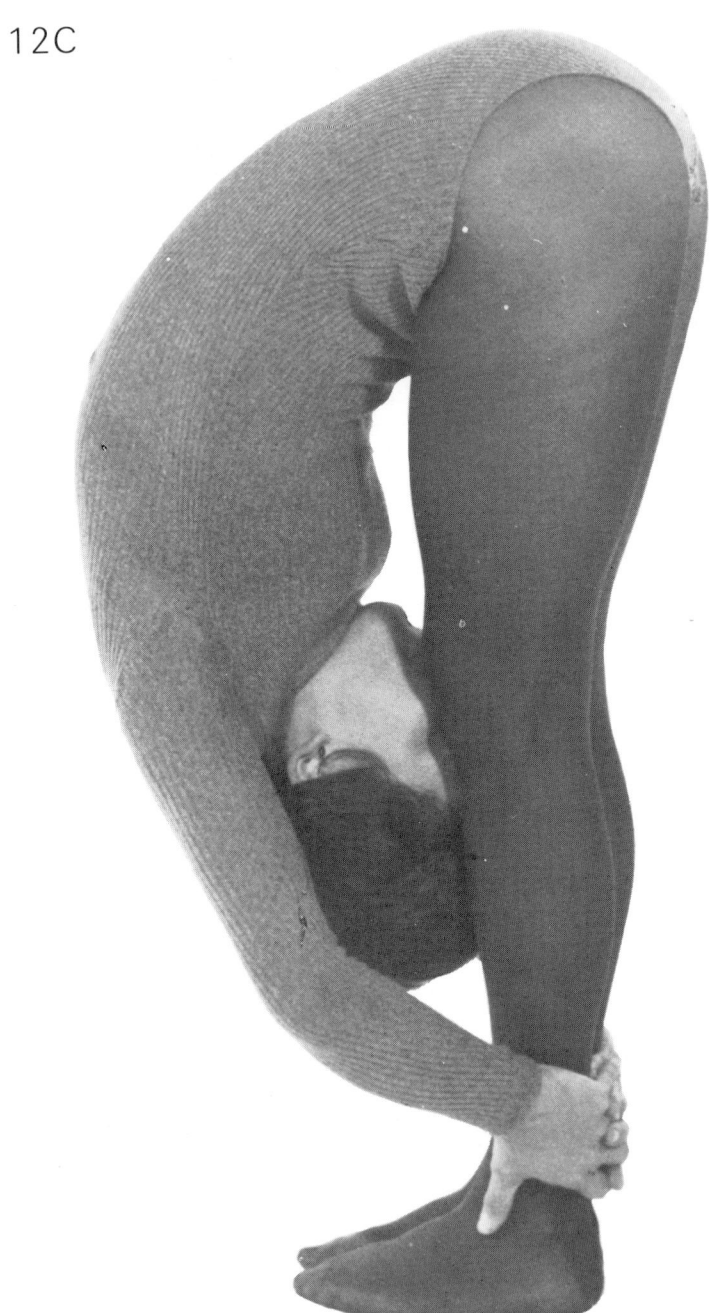

shorter, causing the stooped posture one so often sees in older people.

If you suffer from back trouble, try to keep your knees straight, but don't force or strain. It only matters how each individual eventually exceeds his own limitations, in order to derive the maximum benefit from the Yoga postures.

Practice Technique
Stand erect, bring both arms over your head and inhale deeply. As you bend forward, try to keep your legs straight. Exhale and clasp your hands around your knees. Try to bring your head as close to your knees as you possibly can and hold for five seconds (Fig. 12A).

Release your grip for a moment, and then clasp your hands around your calves, once more bringing your head close to your knees and holding for five seconds (Fig. 12B).

Relax once again and fold your hands around the ankles, bringing your head to the knees and hold for five seconds (Fig. 12C).

Come up, raise your arms high, inhale deeply, and repeat.

Chapter Four

The gentle force and perseverance of Yoga practice is like that of a plant that penetrates through rock and concrete in order to reach the sun.

Yoga to Improve Your Posture

A healthy and correct posture is of the utmost importance to one's appearance. The immediate impact of a beautiful woman can swiftly dissolve when her posture is sloppy or lacks confidence and grace. But one can be struck by the fascinating appearance of a woman who is basically not a beauty but whose charm and regal posture enhance her looks to such an extent that they draw people's interest and attention. Nor ought the importance of posture be ignored by men. For an erect, dynamic appearance indicates the underlying vigour and virility so much admired by all. Posture is as expressive as a dance—it is a joy to watch a body that moves beautifully, with long striding steps, arms that move freely and easily, head held high. It speaks of vitality, personality as well as youth and health.

A correct and graceful posture can create the illusion of being taller; Isadora Duncan, the famous dancer, was a rather short and stocky woman and later on in life even became quite heavy. Nevertheless, she was able to suggest majestic stature, radiate an image of intense beauty and grace, and create vibrations of tremendous power and freedom of the body and the spirit.

It was her conception that movements and expressions originated in the centre of the body. (This is anatomically correct; in Yoga, the navel is called the solar plexus.) These ebullient motions would, as unbroken as the continuous rolling of the waves, stream into the legs, rise into the spine and the arms and translate into the long and flowing expressiveness that became her famous and revolutionary style of dancing.

54

Often the principles and movements of Yoga are incorporated in the dance. In the same way, I believe that we can bring the beauty of Yoga into our daily lives and learn to stand and move with ease, poise, and beauty.

Stand in front of a mirror and look at yourself. Slouching?

Plant the feet firmly on the ground, straighten your back, lift your chest, relax your shoulders, lift up your chin, and don't forget to keep that stomach in. By now you must look like you just swallowed the broomstick. After all, who can possibly remember all these technicalities without keeling over from concentrating on chins, stomachs, a straight back, and what other anatomical details have you.

But since awareness is only half the battle, Yoga will do the other half for you. When you really consistently (by this I mean every day) practise the following exercises, you will see your posture improve dramatically. Especially, when combined with the previous spine postures.

Soon you won't have to concentrate on keeping your back straight or stomach in. Your posture will become erect, your movements free and naturally graceful.

The Tree

If you find it hard to keep your balance in this posture, start out by folding your right leg in such a way that the sole is placed against the inner part of your left thigh. You will find this an easier way to maintain your balance and eventually master the Tree.

Practice Technique

Stand erect. Then slowly shift your weight onto your left leg, and with both hands place your right foot over your left thigh. Bring your hands up over your head, fold the palms together as in prayer, and focus your eyes on one spot in order to maintain a better balance. Keeping your hands together, slowly raise your arms over your head and hold this posture for ten seconds (Fig. 13). Reverse sides and repeat. Gradually increase the hold to forty seconds.

Rishi's Posture

As well as improving posture, Rishi's Posture strengthens the feet and legs remarkably. Try to keep your chin up!

55

13

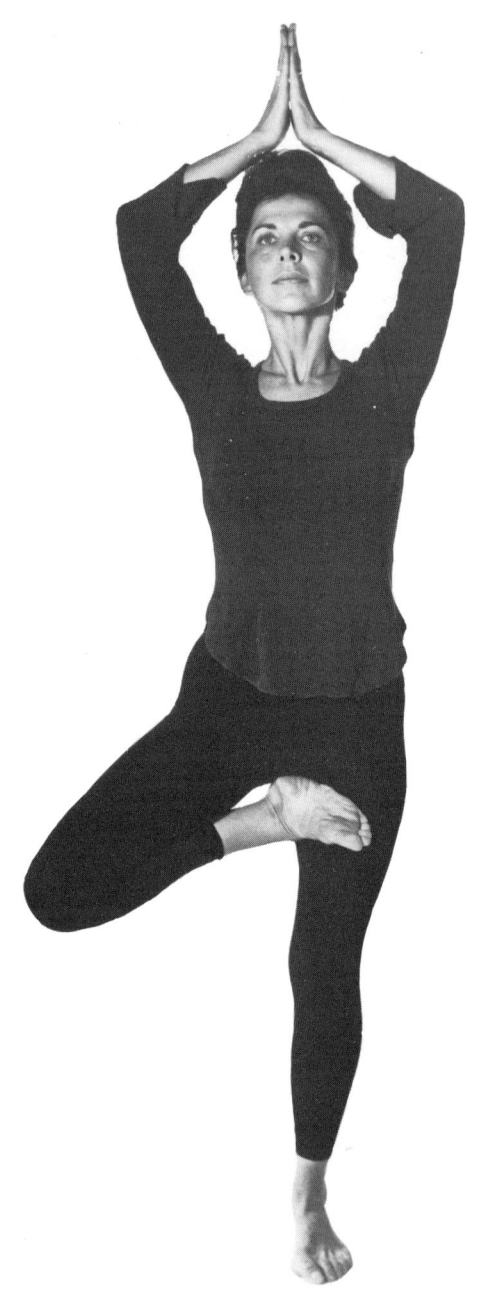

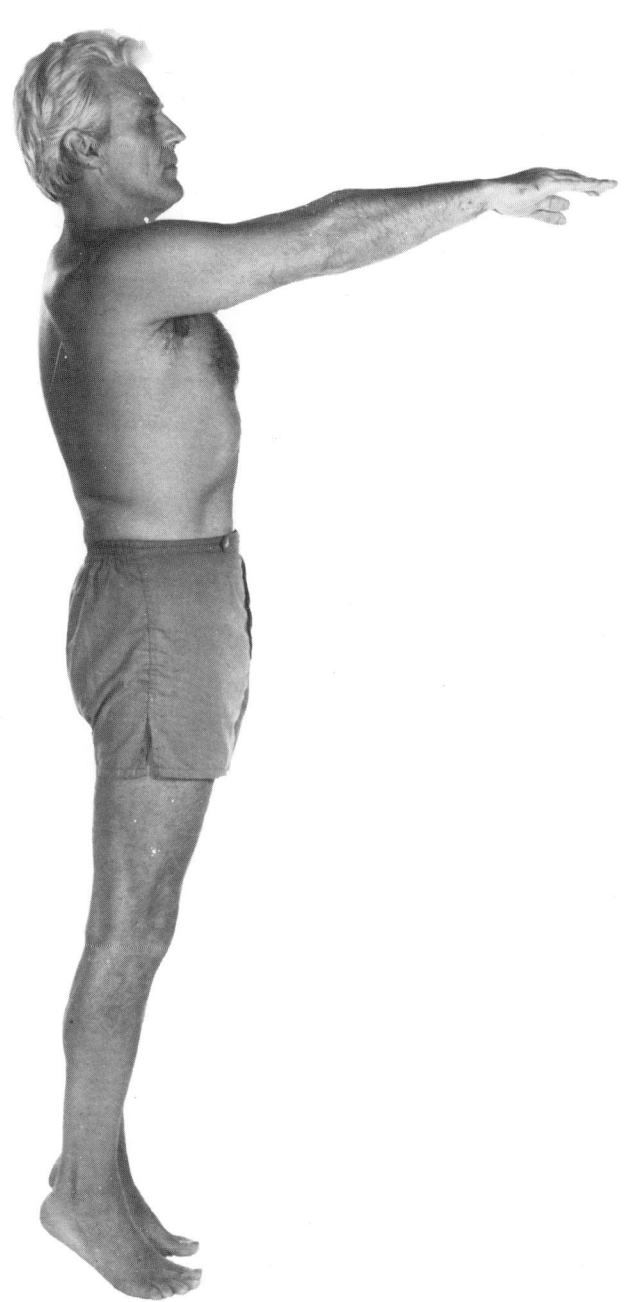

14B

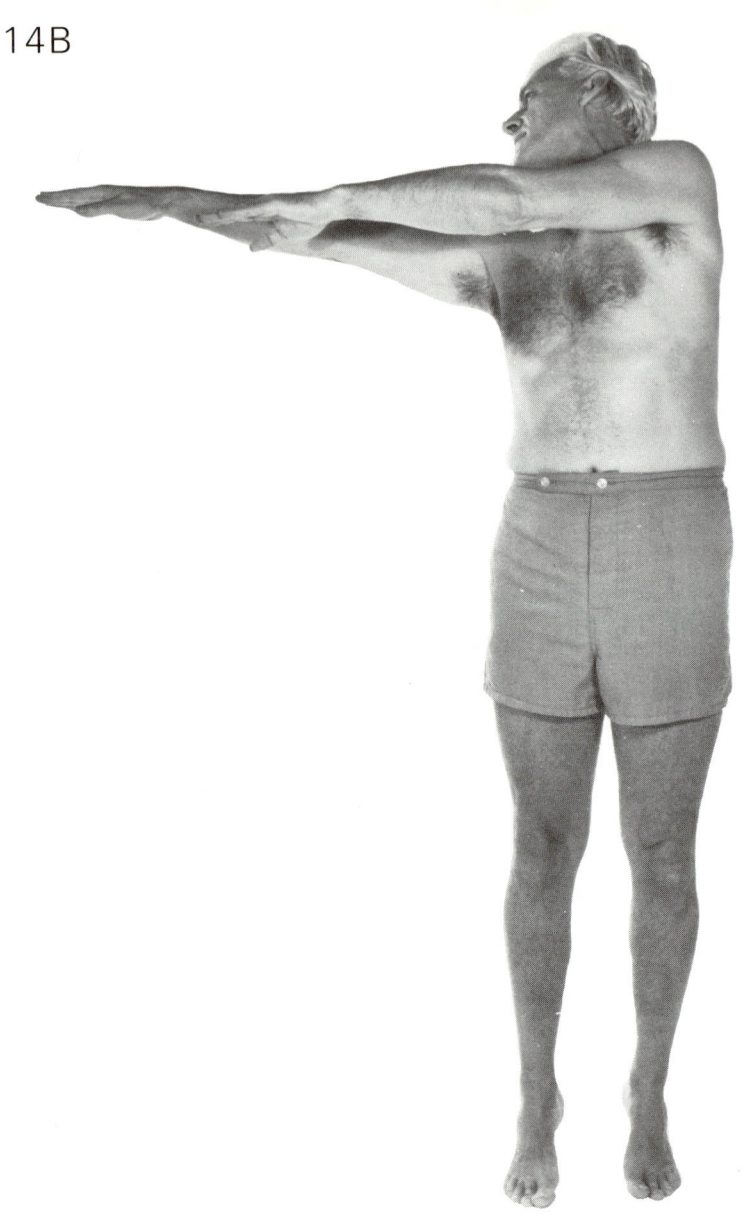

Practice Technique
Stand up on your toes, stretch both arms in front of you palms down, and focus your eyes on the back of your hands (Fig. 14A). Slowly turn your stretched-out arms and the upper part of your body to the right, keeping the lower part in the centre (Fig. 14B).

Maintain this posture for ten seconds, and without coming down onto your heels or lowering the arms, turn to the left side and again hold for ten seconds. Over a period of time increase the duration of the entire posture to forty seconds.

The Dancer's Posture

This beautiful posture creates a wonderful stretch in the body and strengthens the legs and the spine remarkably well. In addition it is an excellent exercise to improve the concentration power and consequently's one's balance.

It stands to reason that the more one raises the arm and the head, the greater the stretch becomes in the body. However, in order to keep a better balance, start off by lifting the arm up slightly and gradually advance by raising the arm and the head way up high.

Practice Technique
Stand erect. Raise your head and bend your right leg backward. Grasp your foot with your right hand and try to press your leg against the buttock. Slowly raise your left arm straight up and hold this posture for ten seconds (Fig. 15A).

Relax and repeat the posture on the opposite side.

After you are able to maintain your balance with ease, proceed by slowly pulling your leg out and upward toward the back of your head (Fig. 15B). Maintain this posture for another ten seconds, gradually to be increased to thirty-five seconds.

Relax and reverse sides.

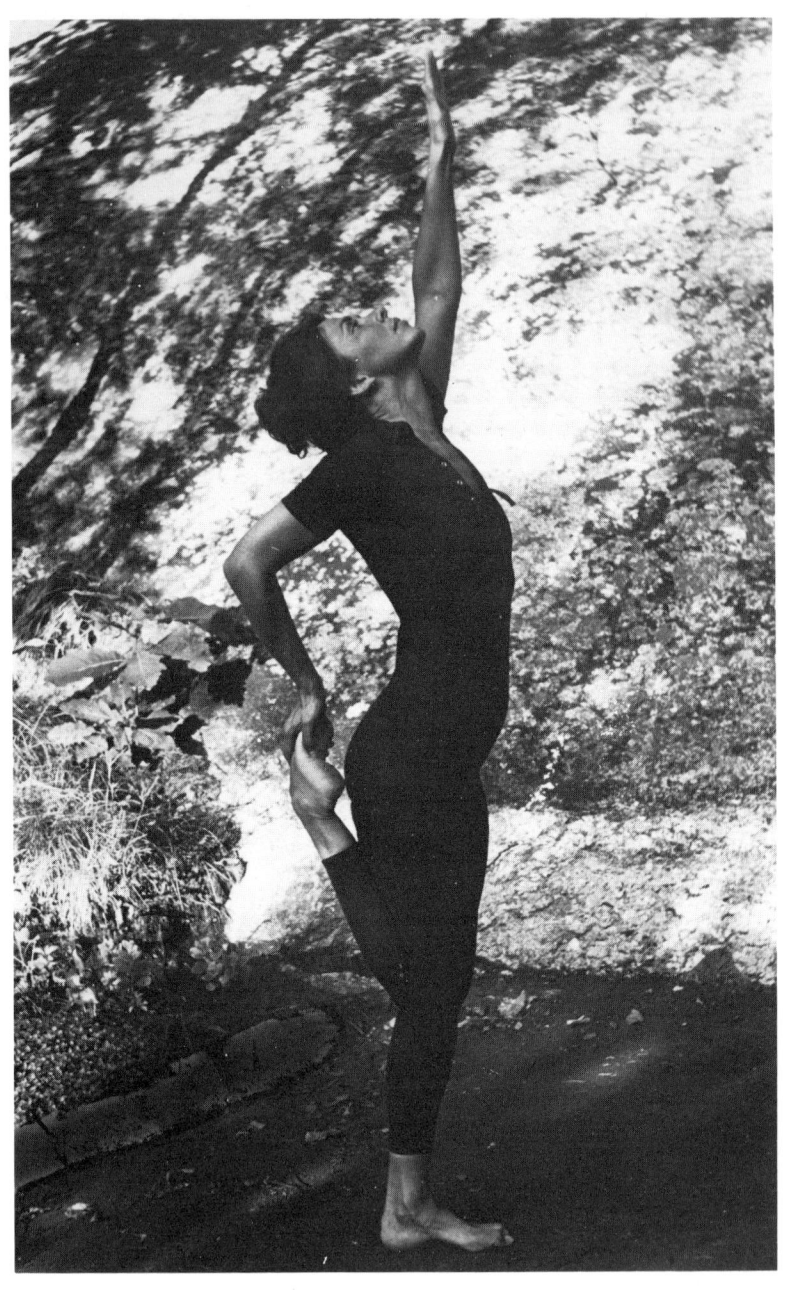

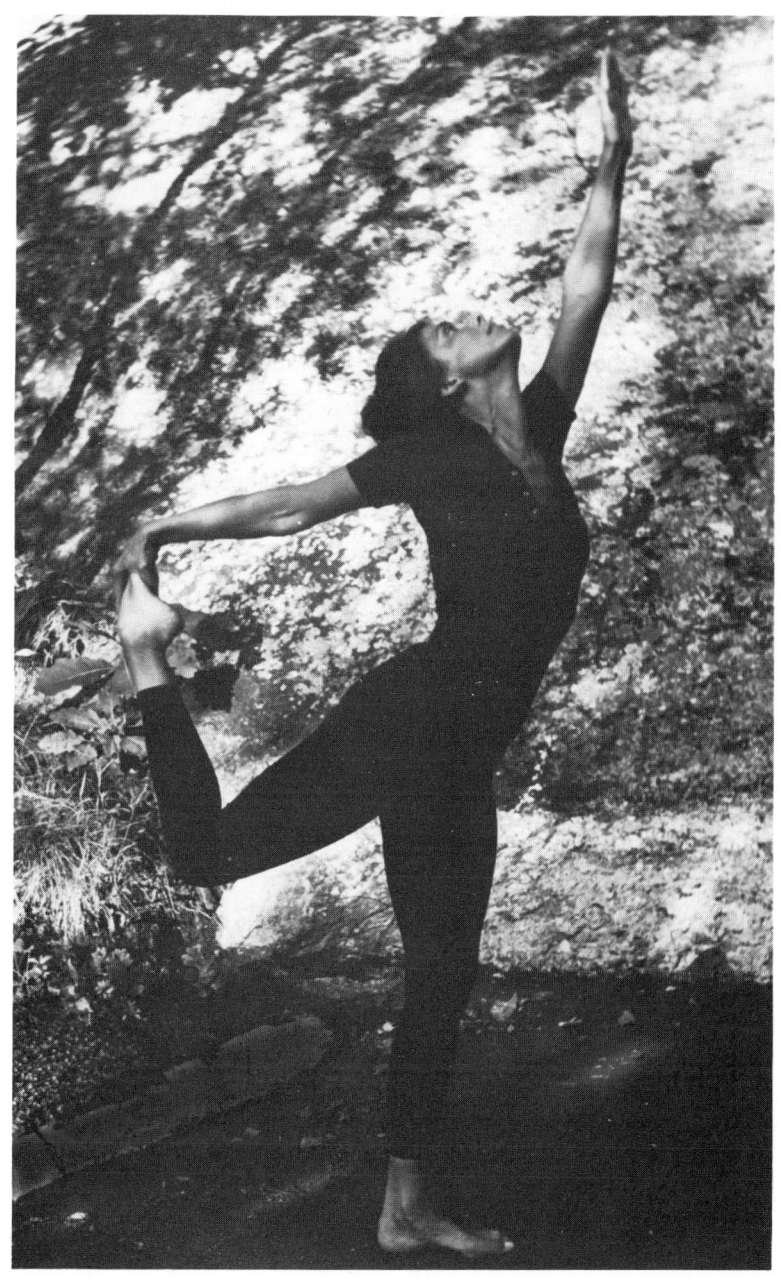

15B

Chapter Five

Yoga generates our awareness of the beauty and magnitude of nature, as well as of the needs, complexity, and potential of man.

Dieting With the Help of Yoga

The nightmare and obsession of almost every man and woman today is being overweight. No one wants to be fat, and let's face it, one does look far more attractive and positively younger after taking off a few extra inches here and there. Not to mention the fact that being overweight endangers one's health.

I can easily give you a diet, but pick up a magazine or go into a bookshop and you'll find innumerable diets published, some old, some new, some of absolute value, some of none whatsoever. I do not believe, for example, in frantic crash diets. Not only are they harmful to our health, but a quick weight loss is just as quickly regained. Furthermore, in order to diet effectively we need enormous determination and will-power. Of course, all of us have moments of defeat. How easy it is to find consolation during one of these ghastly days when everything seems to go wrong, by giving in to that delicious piece of cake that happens to be staring you in the face. But wait—before you sink your teeth into it remember it will give only momentary pleasure (take a carrot or a piece of fruit instead!). Besides, if you stick to your diet maybe next week the scale will show five pounds less. That is far more exciting and certainly of longer lasting pleasure!

In a way, it seems so terribly narcissistic and trivial to be interested in, discuss, and write about diets and looking beautiful, while there are so many terribly urgent causes in our world to be dealt with and solved. But when a person feels unattractive, fat, and clumsy he cannot function to his fullest potential, which is a waste and a loss. When one knows one looks well, one also feels better and more confident and therefore becomes more productive. The Yoga philosophy claims that the body is the temple of the soul and that one should and must be proud of one's body, treating it with love, care, and respect for health as well as aesthetic reasons. What is more beautiful to watch than the body of a child. It moves with tender innocence and natural loveliness. While we are maturing, social inhibitions, personal complexes, and self-consciousness slowly begin to take over and many of us become rigid, uptight, and confined in the use and movements of our body. Consequently, we use far less of our body's total capacity. Slowly our muscles begin to sag and since we burn up far less energy the battle of the bulges has begun.

One cannot and should not stop the process of getting older, but we can and must control the *way* we grow older. So let's get back to the basics. I believe that a high-protein, low-fat, and low-carbohydrate diet is the most sensible and effective. The carbohydrates should not be in the form of sweets or breads, but mostly in the form of vegetables. With this diet, the weight loss will be constant, without that hungry feeling and without danger, especially with a daily intake of vitamins B and C.

And while the pounds are melting off you, it is even more necessary to continue with the Yoga postures, so that together with the weight loss you can regain the youthful figure you once had. First of all there is tightening up to do and at the same time the exercises will redistribute the weight. In myself I have seen a most fantastic change in my figure which I solely attribute to Yoga. My body structure is basically rather pear-shaped—by this I mean all my weight seems to drop into my bottom and thighs. Nothing but starvation would ever change this, but instead of engaging in such drastic measures, Yoga has taken off those extra inches.

Once you have reached your desired weight, eat sensibly. Weigh yourself regularly, and don't ever let more than five pounds creep up. But if you do gain five pounds or so, start immediately with the cited diet again until you are back to where you were before, which should not take more than a week or two. And continue to exercise—that combined with proper diet is the secret of staying slim forever!

In the following chapters, I will give Yoga postures that will firm, tighten, and reduce each part of the body.

Chapter Six

Stamina of body and strength of spirit are the vital requirements of survival.

The Neck and Chin

The neck is the pedestal on which the head rests like a piece of sculpture. It is also the spot where tension often seems to gather, and I hate to remind you, one of the areas where age announces itself. But don't despair, we can hold the demon of age back a little longer. Let's find out the reason why age opens its attack on this particular area. I believe it is because the muscles under the chin and in the neck receive the least amount of use, and therefore, lose their elasticity more rapidly. So, obviously, the answer is to keep them moving and stretching, and fortunately the Yoga postures put great emphasis on this whole region of muscles.

Since I just accused age of being a demon, there is something I would like to clarify. Because we are living in a youth-oriented society, many of us seem to consider ourselves on the decline when we get close to forty, and some past this traumatic number prefer not to count altogether. This is a self-defeating and unjust attitude, and women in particular seem susceptible to it. A woman in her forties is in her prime and has a lot to offer—poise, intelligence, and personality can make her a more interesting, secure, and complete person, providing she is aware of these powers and uses her assets, rather than crumbling under the pressure of this Western youth-myth and the appearance of a few wrinkles. We have earned those! We are alive, and life cannot pass by and leave us untouched. It is what makes us grow and develop as a person and gives us character and personality.

But even when we accept the normal process of ageing and learn to live with our wrinkles, it does not mean that we should become negligent of our body and let our appearance go.

64

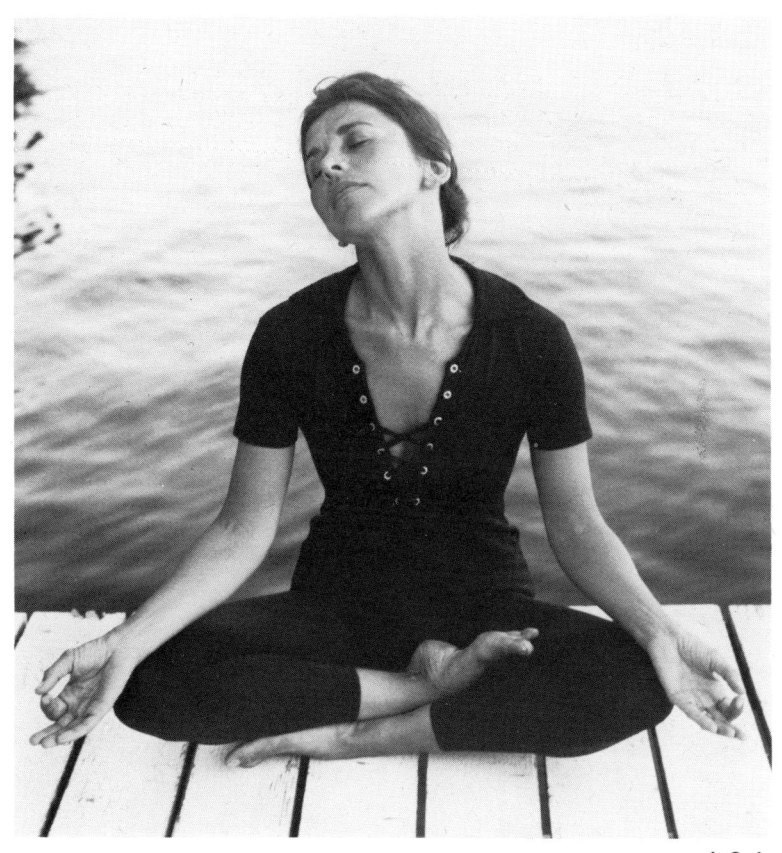

We can and should continue to stay trim, limber, and fit, but it does take a little more time, effort, and sacrifice. Do keep your body firm and tight, if only out of self-respect!

I shall give you several neck and chin exercises which you can practise at any given moment, such as when you are on the phone, on the bus, or at the next PTA meeting.

In previous chapters there are postures such as the Cobra (Fig. 6B) and the Dancer's Posture (Fig. 15A) which are also effective for the chin and neck.

The Neck Stretch

After you have learned this posture you will see that one can hold and repeat it at any time and almost any place and as often as one wishes.

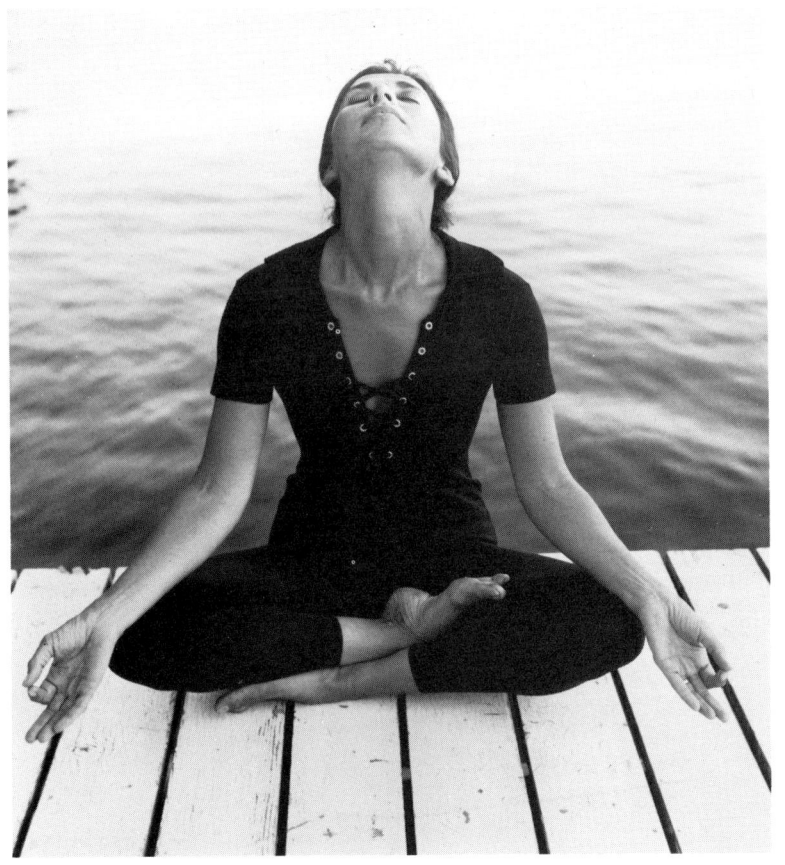

Practice Technique

Sit in your most comfortable Lotus position. Slowly roll your head to the right, making sure to keep your body in the centre and your shoulders way down. In order to derive an ultimate stretch in the chin and the neck muscles, protrude your chin slightly as well. Close your eyes and hold this position for thirty seconds (Fig. 16A).

Now slowly roll your head all the way to the back. Again, body centred, shoulders down, chin out (Fig. 16B). Hold for thirty seconds.

Repeat on the left, and after thirty seconds roll your head all the way forward. After several seconds repeat this entire exercise in a counterclockwise direction.

Chapter Seven

The slow intensity of Yoga postures expands into a total awareness of the body.

The Chest

The female breast has been celebrated in poetry and song, its beauty symbolized in every form and school of art. For here lies the heart, wellspring of affection, source of life and cradle of the infant, as well as the irresistible seducer of men! In the male of the species the outthrust chest becomes the representation of dignity and strength.

Will we carry our precious vessels low, half-hidden on a concave chest, or proudly extend our bosom, regardless of what its size might be! (This meekly stated by your bereft AA-cup authoress.) It is important to keep the pectoral muscles strong and elastic, for it is the weakening of these muscles that will cause the unfortunate sagging of the breasts.

The following Yoga postures will strengthen these muscles and are especially recommended during and after nursing, or while undergoing significant weight loss through dieting.

The Swan

As I pointed out in the chapter on the five fundamental Yoga postures, the Swan is an extremely beneficial posture for the entire body. It works out the chin, neck, arms, chest, spine, abdomen, pelvis, legs, and feet, and is exhilarating to do.

Practice Technique
Sit in your comfortable Lotus position. Clasp your hands together behind you, tighten your abdomen, and raise your hands as high as possible, keeping your chin way up (Fig. 17A). Hold this posture for a minimum of fifteen seconds, gradually increasing the duration of the hold.

The Camel and Child's Poses
Practice Technique
Kneel down, toes touching the floor and your back straight. Take hold of the heel of your right foot with the corresponding hand. Do the same on the left side.

Slowly lean all the way back, bending your head back as well (Fig. 17B). At first hold this position for five seconds and gradually increase the time to twenty-five seconds. Slowly come out of this position, and to counteract the extreme concave bend of the spine come forward in the Child's Pose in order to relax this way for several moments (Fig. 17C).

17A

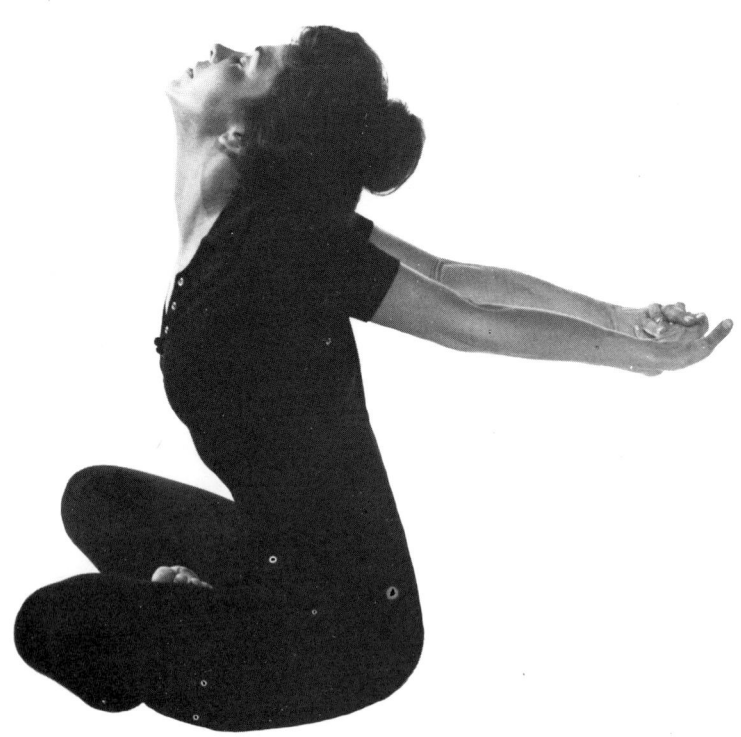

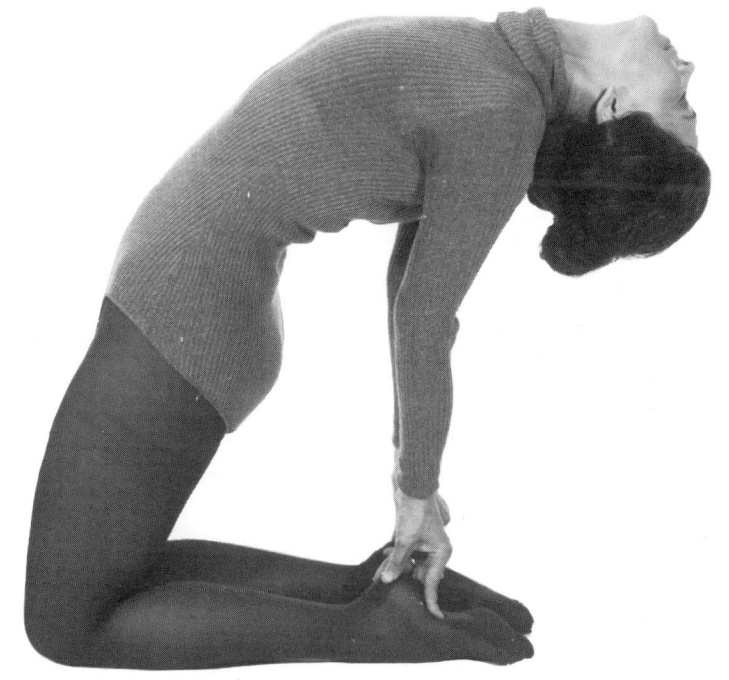

17B

17C

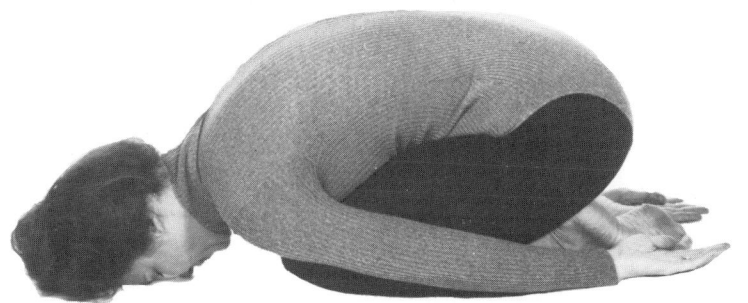

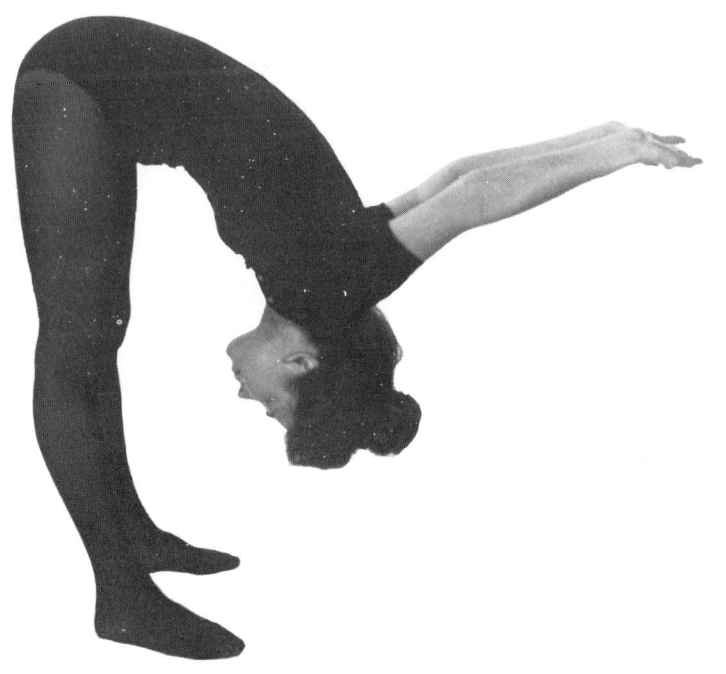

18A

The Chest Expansion

Although this posture is called the Chest Expansion, it does much more than just that. Its convex posture limbers and stretches the entire spine, while the legs can get quite a workout as well if you remember not to bend the knees!

Practice Technique
Stand straight with your feet slightly apart. Clasp both hands together behind your back, inhale deeply, and simultaneously lift your arms as high as you are able to. As you start to bend forward, exhale and continue to keep your arms up high (Fig. 18A). Bend as far forward as possible. Relax your neck, breathe deeply, and hold the posture for ten seconds.

Now bend toward your right leg and try to bring your forehead closely to the knee (Fig. 18B), hold for five seconds and turn the body toward the left side in order to reverse and to repeat the posture.

Return the body to the centre, arms up high at all times, the neck relaxed, and start to come up in an extremely slow tempo.

Tighten the muscles in the thighs, abdomen, buttocks, midriff, and raise your head. Inhale deeply, hold for five seconds, and relax.

18B

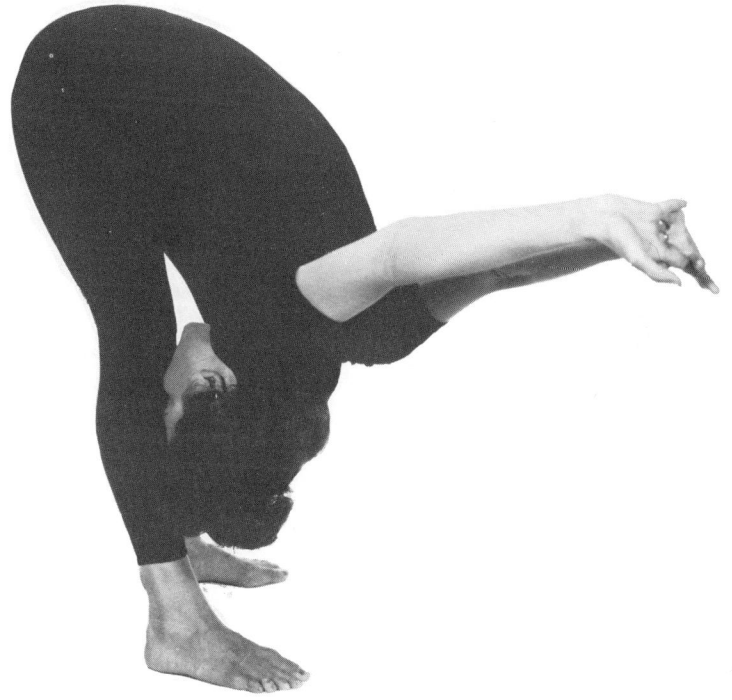

Chapter Eight

My hands reached out, for I sensed your need and loneliness, and when we touched I felt your lifestream flowing into mine. The tender beauty of that moment floated in the air as fragile as a multicoloured bubble, and I could not speak, afraid that even words might break its crystal loveliness.

The Arms and Hands

The hands are an extension of our inner self, for they become the instrument of our mind and emotions. They can destroy as well as create great beauty, forming fists in hate or touching and reaching out in love. The movements and gestures of arms and hands can be stronger and more expressive than words.

Of course, the dance is the ultimate example of the unlimited emotions our bodies can express. Why not take some of the grace and beauty of dance and incorporate it into our daily lives?

I mentioned before and will mention again how very important a good posture is. Posture can be improved by moving the arms with long and flowing motions—and do remember that arms begin at the shoulder and should be used as such, for the effect is far more regal and dramatic.

Sometimes it becomes easier to communicate when our hands gently emphasize the words we speak (this certainly is essential for me, not always having that Dutch dictionary around!).

The Yoga Seal
It can be difficult at first to bend all the way forward as this posture suggests, but try to come down as far as you comfortably can and you will derive exactly the same benefit from the postures as someone whose body is more limber through longer experience with Yoga. Gradually increase the time, stay with it, and who knows what miracles might happen!!

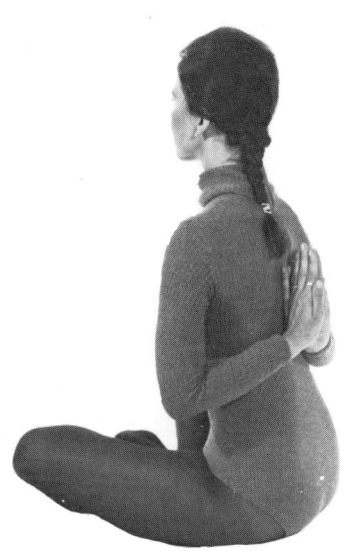

19A

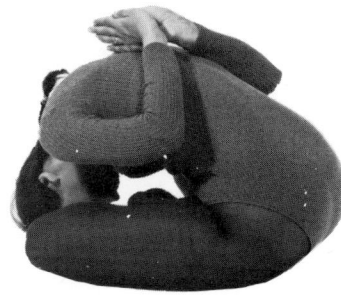
19B

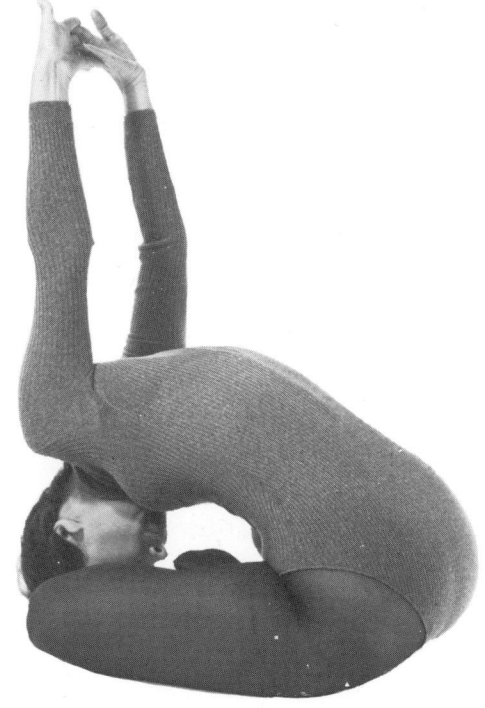
19C

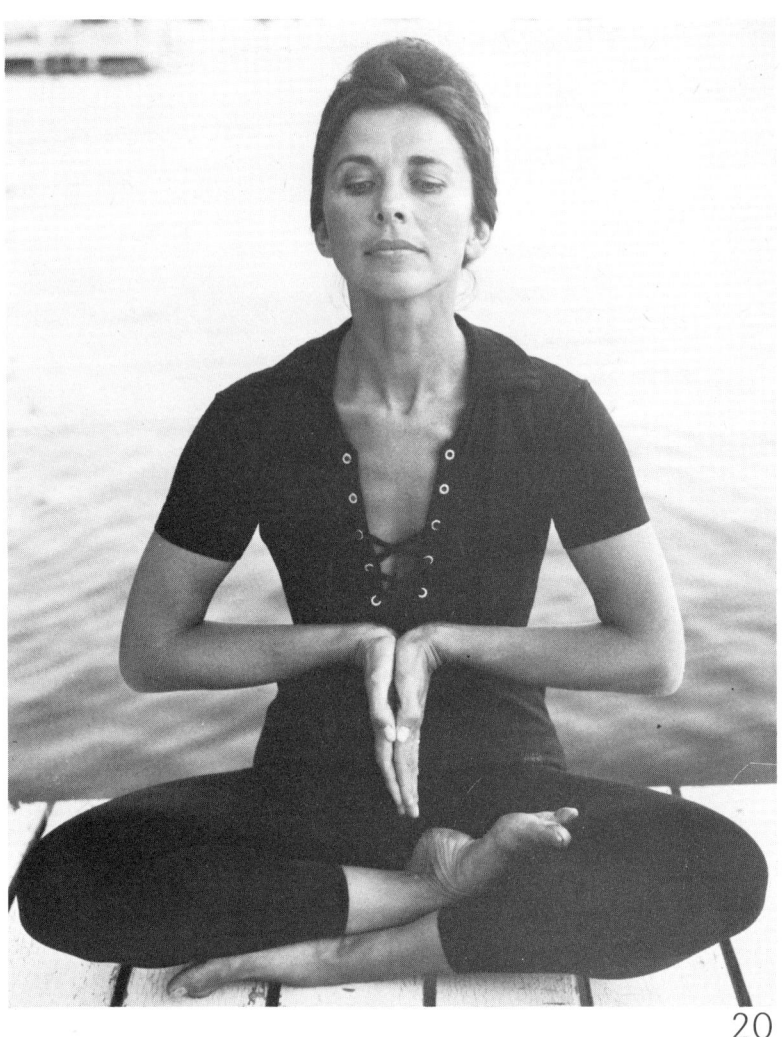

20

Practice Technique

Sit in your most comfortable Lotus position. Bring your hands behind you and press your palms together. Throw the shoulders back, while slowly turning your hands inward and then upward so that the outside of your small fingers touch your back (Fig. 19A). Inhale, then exhale and bend forward, relaxing your neck and holding this posture for five seconds (Fig. 19B).

Bring your hands down and turn them out so your fingers

point away from your body. Intertwine your fingers and clasp your hands together. Raise your arms as high as possible (Fig. 19C). Hold for five seconds. Now slowly draw your spine up straight, which will bring your arms down to about the middle of your back. (You will notice that you have ended in the Swan pose.) Inhale deeply, relax.

The Vibration Posture
This is an excellent exercise for firming the upper arms and strengthening the pectoral muscles.

Practice Technique
Sit in your most comfortable Lotus position. Remember to keep your chin up and your shoulders down at all times.

Press the hands so firmly together that you feel the arms vibrate strenuously (Fig. 20). Do this for fifteen seconds, and then repeat three more times.

Chapter Nine

And on her lover's arm she leant
and round her waist she felt it fold
and far across the hills they went
in that new world which is the old.
   (from 'THE DEPARTURE'—Tennyson)

The Waist

How utterly romantic! Perhaps we all sometimes dream of having a torrid love affair and imagine ourselves wandering through the hills, our lover's arm wrapped around our waist! Just in case, we ought to make sure we have a waist that an arm can fit around. So let's practise the postures.

The Waistroll

Make sure your shoulders, arms, and hands remain on the floor during this entire exercise as that will create a greater stretch in the waist and the thoracic area of the spine.

Practice Technique

Lie down on your back and place your hands, palms up, next to your shoulders. Using only your stomach muscles, pull both knees up and press them against your abdomen. Keeping your knees and feet close together, very slowly roll them to the right and at the same time roll your head to the left (Fig. 21A). Hold this position for five seconds. Now roll your legs slowly to the left and your head to the right (Fig. 21B). Again hold for five seconds. Repeat on each side four more times. Next bring both legs to the centre, raise them into a vertical position, and take twenty seconds to lower then. Relax and breathe deeply.

The Triangle

In order to perform the extreme stretch you can achieve through this posture, make sure you bend your body in an absolutely sideward and not in a partly forward position. And remember to keep the legs straight.

76

Practice Technique

Stand erect, arms at your sides, feet apart, and raise your arms sideward to shoulder level. Look at your right hand, and begin bending from the waist, bringing the upper part or your body to the left. Make sure your right arm is as close to your head as possible in order to create an ultimate stretch in the waist

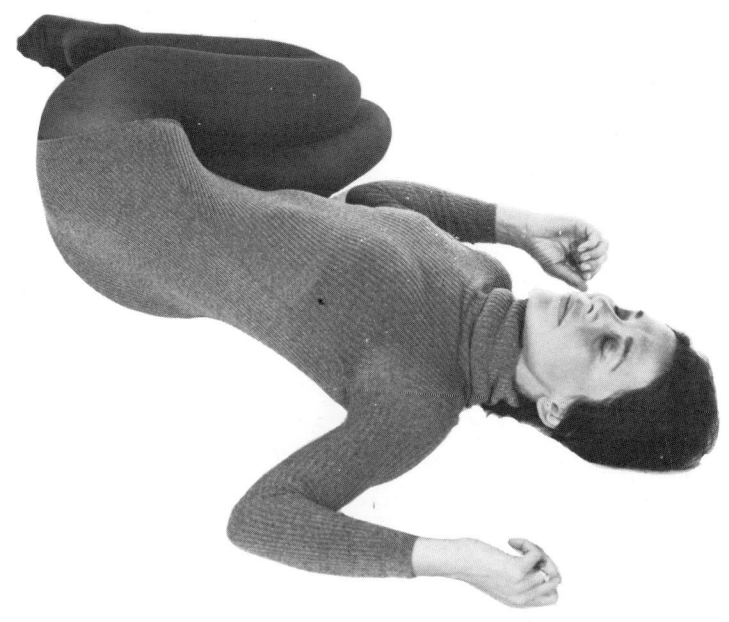

21A

21B

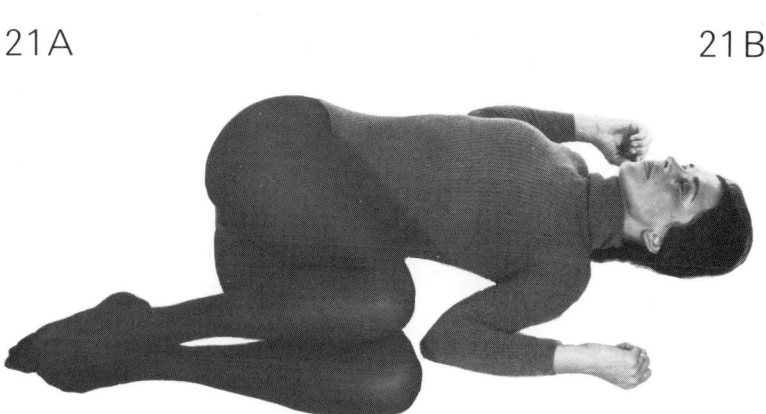

and hip. Hold for fifteen seconds and slowly return your body to the centre. Repeat the Triangle in the opposite direction (Fig. 22).

Gradually increase the time to thirty-five seconds.

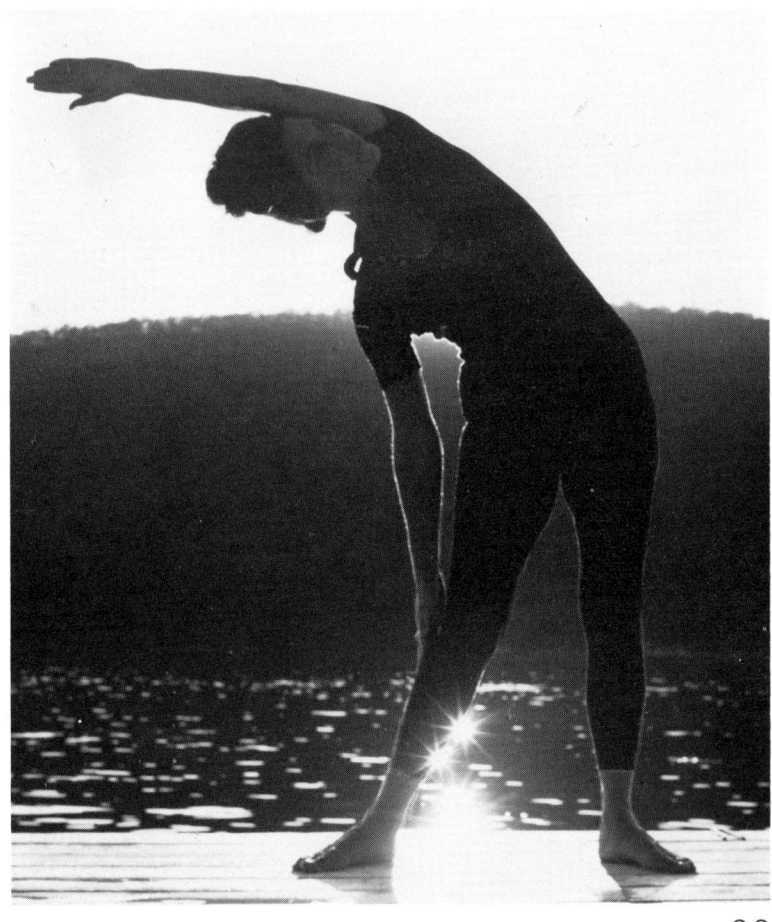

22

Chapter Ten

Yoga is received by the body as gently as a flower is unfolded by the sunlight.

The Abdomen

At the mentioning of the word abdomen, do we lower our eyes in dismay to make sure our own belly is not sticking out too much? Certainly it is a constant battle to get and keep the abdomen flat.

It seems as we get older the abdominal muscles do not function as much in our daily activities, and therefore, they deteriorate rapidly. What we often accuse of being 'a fat tummy' may actually be the sad result of sagging, flabby muscles.

All of us are aware that that isn't the most aesthetically flattering image one can project, but unknown to many is the fact that the abdominal musculature functions as the chief support of our back! It therefore is of vital importance to exercise and strengthen the abdominal muscles. In addition, the abdomen gives shelter to the solar plexus, a most complex centre of nerve cells that controls the activities and functioning of the abdominal organs. Many Yoga postures will activate and stimulate the working of these organs which may have become sluggish and weak because of a sedentary way of life.

The Abdominal Contraction

I consider the following exercise one of the most essential in Yoga. Not only will it stimulate and invigorate the functioning of the abdominal organs, but it will help you gain tremendous control over the abdominal muscles, resulting in much stronger and tighter muscles of the midriff and the abdomen.

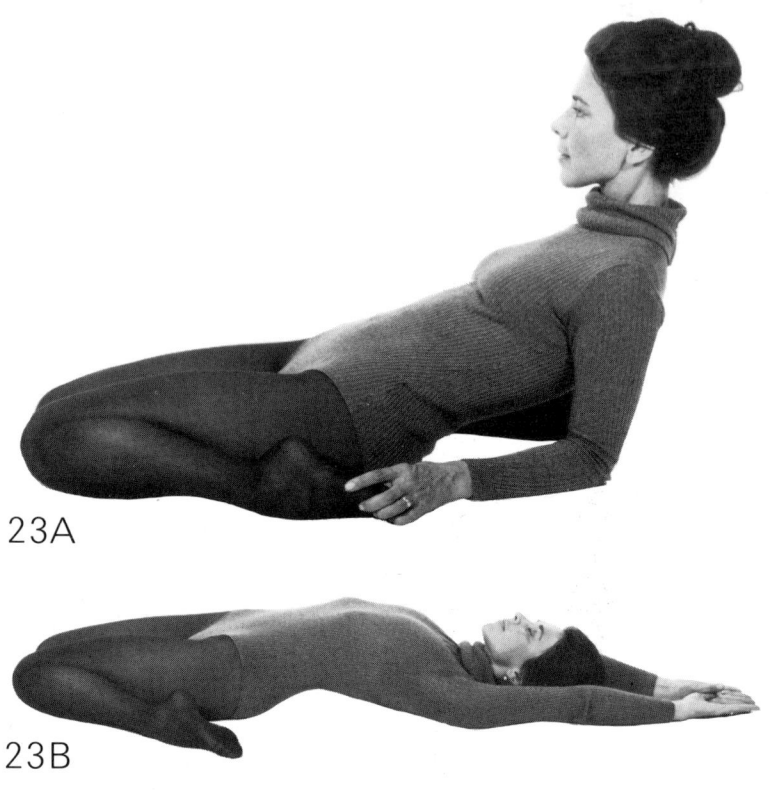

23A

23B

Practice Technique

Sit in any position that is most comfortable to you although this exercise can also be practised in a standing or even a lying down position.

Place your hands on your knees and sit up straight.

Pull in the muscles of your abdomen as far as you can and hold for three seconds. At the count of four, push the muscles as far out as possible. Immediately draw the muscles in as hard as you can and hold for three counts. Again at the count of four, push your abdomen out and repeat eight more contractions and releases in a slow and even tempo. That comprises one round. Relax, breathe deeply, and continue for two more rounds of ten contractions each.

Since this is a rather strenuous exercise, work very gradually up to fifty contractions per round for three rounds, making sure to breathe deeply and relax between each round.

The Ultimate Body Stretch

This posture gives the entire body an ultimate stretch, stimulates the digestive system, and improves the functioning of the intestines. In addition, it strengthens the muscles in the abdomen, thighs, and feet. Some people might find this posture extremely difficult. But remember never to strain the body or force a posture. Practise by simply trying to sit between both feet for as long as you can; perhaps one day you will master this one.

Practice Technique
Kneel on the floor, your feet apart, and lower your buttocks between your feet to the floor. Holding onto each foot, first lean back on the right elbow, then on both elbows (Fig. 23A), and gently lie down flat on your back.

Continue to lie flat for five seconds. After practising this posture for a while, advance by bringing your arms way over the head (Fig. 23B) and stretching the entire body. Stay in this position for as long as you are comfortable, and continue to breathe deeply by extending the abdomen while inhaling, and contracting when exhaling, feeling the navel press against the spine. This is the so-called abdominal Yoga breathing. This technique allows the lungs to fill up to their fullest capacity.

Come out of the position in reverse order, then bend forward into the Child's Pose (Fig. 17B) where you will relax for several moments.

The Boat

Lie down on your back with your arms next to your body. Simultaneously raise your trunk and your legs off the floor and place your arms on the side of your knees (Fig. 24). Maintain this position for fifteen seconds, to be gradually increased to forty.

The Upward Leg Pull

This is a tricky one. At first, you will find it rather difficult, if not impossible to maintain your balance while keeping your legs straight. Perhaps it will be easier for you in the beginning to grasp your calves or ankles, and eventually, after enough practice, your big toes. If done correctly, this position will

81

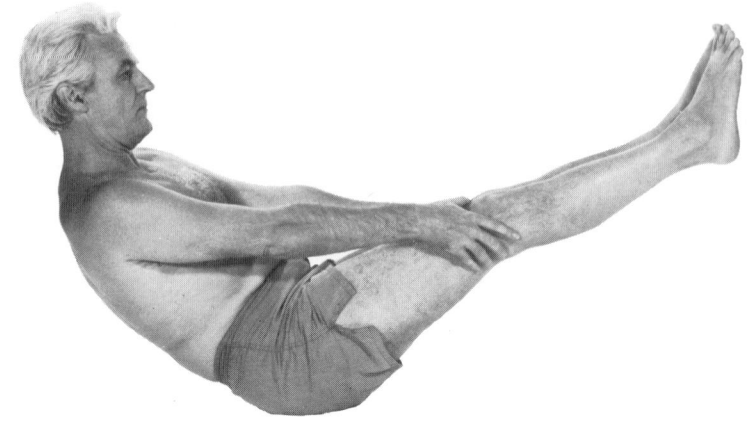

24

strengthen the hamstring tendons as well as the muscles in back of the knees.

Have fun with this one.

Practice Technique
Sit down with your legs stretched out straight in front of you. Bend your knees and grasp your big toes. Now slowly raise your legs, straightening them out at the same time (Fig. 25).

Hold for five seconds, gradually increasing the time to thirty-five seconds.

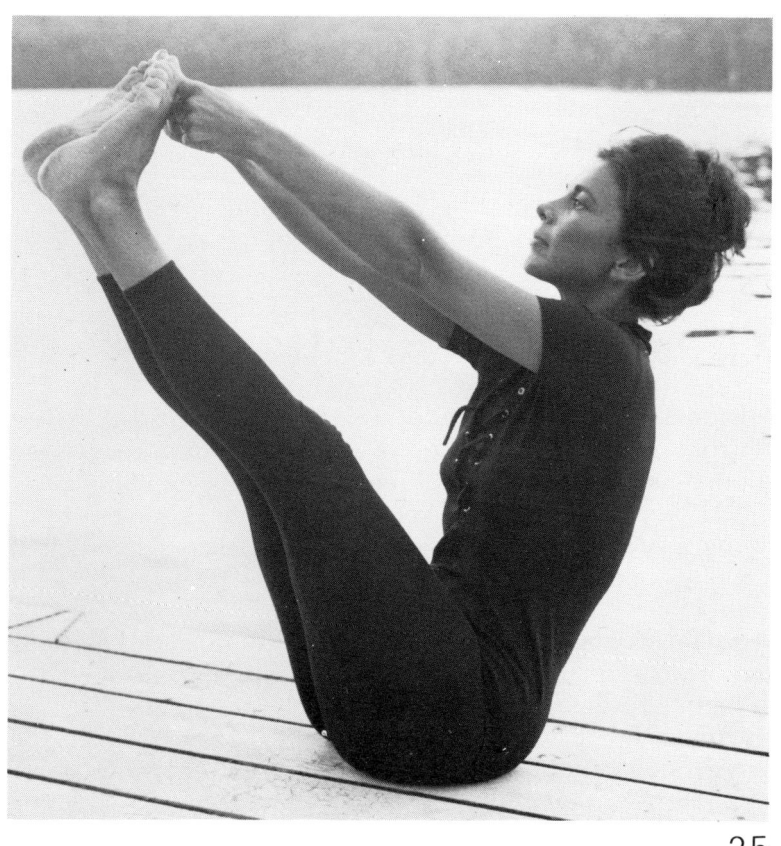

25

Chapter Eleven

Yoga tries to establish a harmonious balance between the body and the mind.

The Hips and Buttocks

Fortunately we are saved from seeing ourselves from the back, for that sight might cause quite a shock. Modern times have spoiled us with comfort and luxury. Instead of walking a few blocks, we take the car, we spend many hours sitting in front of the TV, and ingenious appliances have taken over much of the physical labour that once kept us going from morning till night.

One pays a price for everything in life and in this particular case the price is often infamous middle-age spread— drooping bottoms, oversized hips, flabby thighs.

Obviously we will continue to drive cars and watch TV (sitting down, not standing up), and I would hardly suggest that you get rid of your washing machine. But at least let us try to keep our muscles firm and tight. For instance, use every opportunity to walk, as walking is one of the most simple and healthful exercises—besides, it puts us so much more in touch with life around us.

And, of course, one's heritage—in my case, Dutch—never belies itself. Holland is a country with an infinite sky, a history many times greater than its size, a spring that explodes into a multitude of brilliant colours, and millions of people riding bicycles almost everywhere they go. So I suggest you ride a bicycle, not only as a form of recreation, but as a means of transportation. It is fast (sensational in the rush hours!), economical, healthy, and lots of fun. And if more people ride bicycles, it will not only alleviate our ghastly traffic jams, but it will play a small part in our effort to solve the air pollution crisis. That is a problem which concerns everybody, for this is our planet—let each of us strive to preserve it.

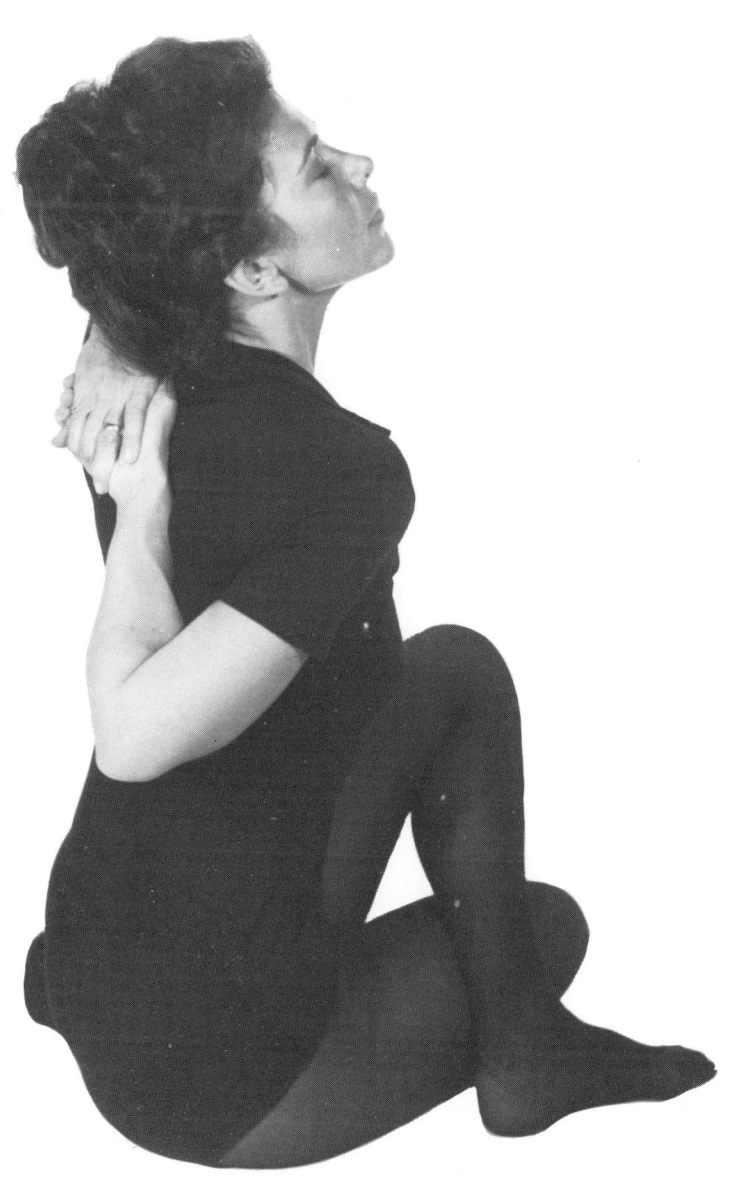

26A

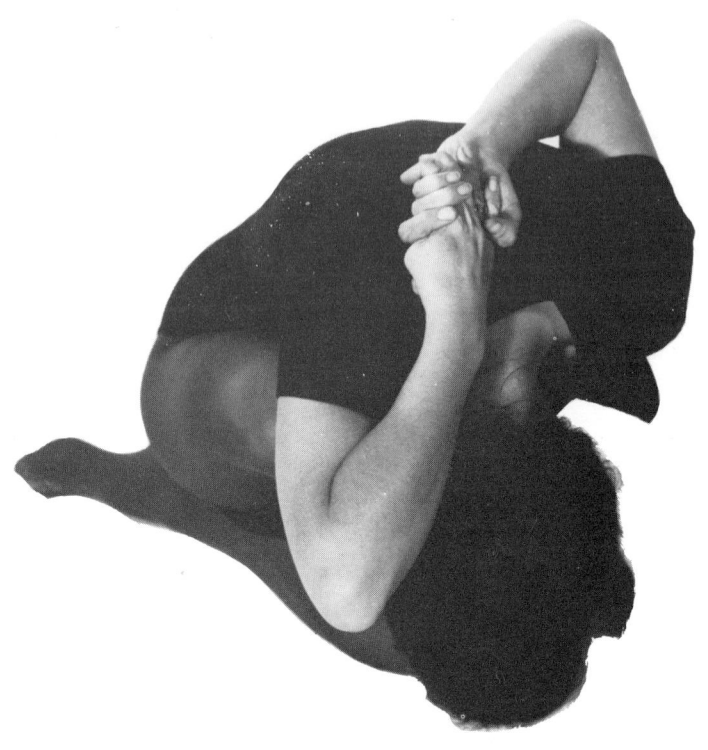

26B

In addition to these vigorous activities, we can take inches
off our hips and reduce our buttocks to a more moderate size
by consistent practice of the following Yoga postures.

The Warrior
This exercise works out the shoulders, arms, and hands—and
it firms the muscles in the thighs as well!

It becomes especially important as a preventive exercise
against bursitis and the formation of calcium deposits in the
shoulders.

Practice Technique
Sit on the floor with both legs stretched out in front of you.
Bend your right leg and place your right sole against your left

thigh as close to the groin as possible. Bend your left knee, take the ankle in both hands and bring the leg over your folded right leg. Place the sole of your left foot on the floor.

Now bring your left arm over your left shoulder and down your back, and the right arm under your right shoulder and up your back. Try to bring both hands as close together as possible, ultimately clasping them together (Fig. 26A). Keep your chin way up high and hold this pose for ten seconds. Slowly bend forward as far as possible without strain and hold another ten seconds (Fig. 26B). Come back up, relax your arms and legs, and repeat the posture on the opposite side.

The Pelvic Stretch
Sit on the floor and stretch both legs in front of you. Place the palms of your hands on the floor behind you. Lift the entire pelvic area upward while keeping your body straight (Fig. 27).

Hold for five seconds and gradually increase to twenty seconds.

The Half Locust
This is a rather strenuous posture and should not be practised during the menstrual period, nor by people suffering from hernia, high blood pressure, or serious back trouble.

Practice Technique
Lie down on your stomach, resting your chin on the floor. Place your arms alongside the body and form your hands into fists.

27

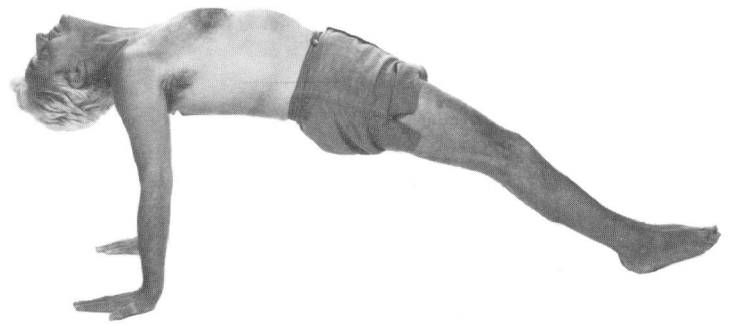

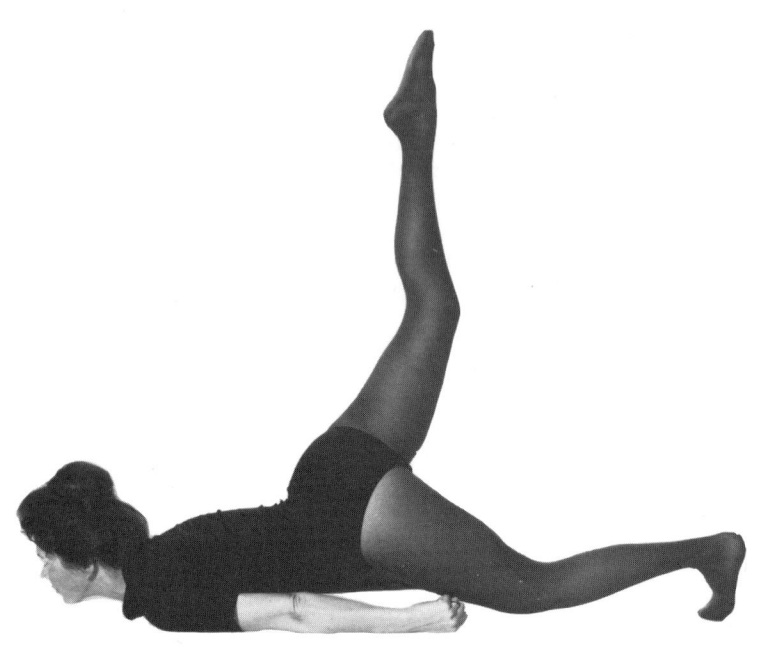

28A

Arch your left leg by leaning on the knee and toes, inhale, and slowly raise your right leg as high as you can (Fig. 28A). Your weight should be resting on your chin, chest, and arms. Hold for five seconds, then slowly lower your leg. Close your eyes and relax completely until your heartbeat has become regular.

Reverse sides and repeat. Gradually increase your holding time until you can retain this posture for as long as twenty-five seconds.

Full Locust

After you are able to hold the Half Locust for twenty-five seconds, progress by starting to practise the Full Locust.

To achieve a great support, lie on your right side, interlock your fingers, and then roll your body onto your stomach. Rest your chin on the floor, inhale deeply, stiffen your whole body, and slowly raise both legs off the floor (Fig. 28B).

88

Again, your weight rests on the chin, chest, and especially your arms. Hold for five seconds, close your eyes, and relax completely until your heartbeat has become regular.

Gradually increase the time to fifteen seconds.

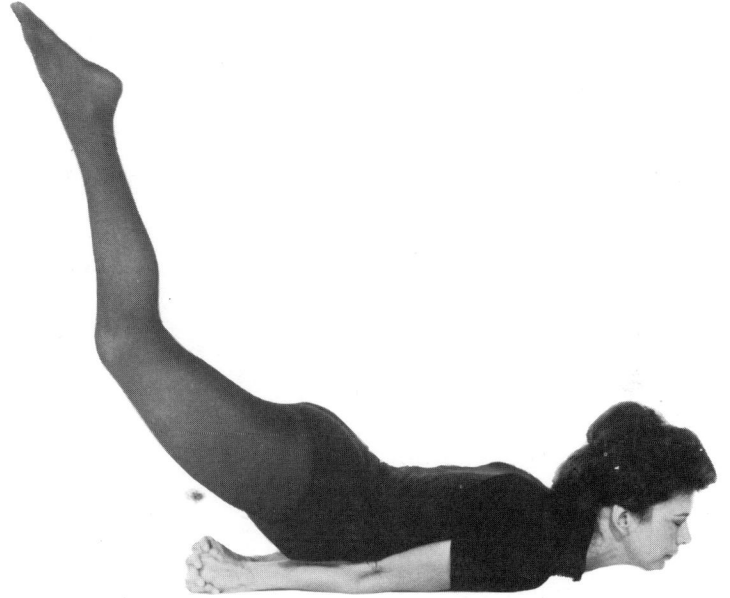

28B

Chapter Twelve

The movements of Yoga, interwoven with the beauty of a dance, teach the body control heightened by grace.

The Legs and Feet

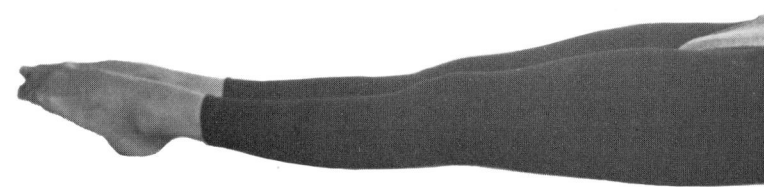

Our legs take us to faraway places, climb over the highest mountains, dance through the night, and help us escape from danger. But it is not only for practical reasons that we should keep them strong and limber, for the shape of our legs and the way we move them have an enormous effect on our overall appearance. The movements of legs can be airy and lyrical or excitingly sensuous and earthy.

Let us once more return to Isadora Duncan, who made her pupils practise the art of walking for hours on end with motions based on the beautiful movements of the Lippizzaner horses, whose famous walk has been described as 'floating in air.'

29B

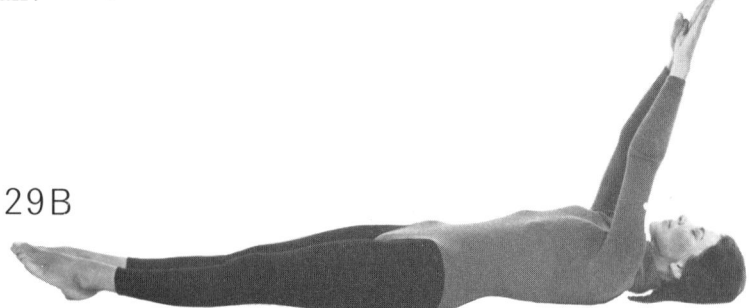

Now we mere mortals can hardly expect to float in the air, but we should learn to move our legs from the hips in long and flowing rhythms, lightly carrying an erect and graceful body.

The following Yoga postures will help you to strengthen your legs (especially tendons and ligaments you never even knew you possessed), reduce your thighs, work out stiffness in knees, ankles, and feet. And, just as important, these Yoga postures will be of aid in preventing or relieving those feared and despised varicose veins. Varicose veins are caused by a

29A

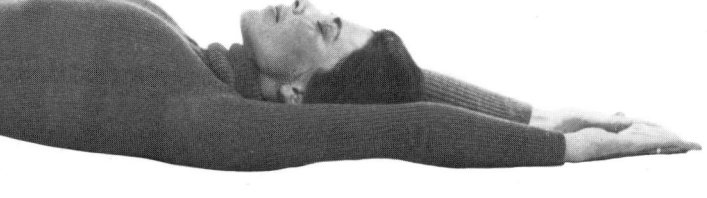

loss of elasticity of the veins. This can be compared to a rubberband that has lost its spring. The Yoga postures strengthen the surrounding muscles and connective tissues, adding support around these veins and therefore protecting the veins from losing their resilience.

Apart from the specified postures, I strongly advise the Shoulderstand and Headstand—in the stages you can comfortably and safely do—for they are particularly effective in stimulating the blood circulation in the legs. Increased blood circulation can be most helpful in avoiding the danger of arthritis, as well as in keeping the skin tight and healthy, and preventing, to a great extent, the unpleasant cramping of the feet and toes.

The Leg Pull

For this posture do not bend the knees, and don't get discouraged when you are unable to reach your toes. And if it is difficult at first to come up from a reclining position, start this posture from a sitting position. By gradually increasing the holding time to thirty seconds, you will find yourself getting closer to your toes all the time. Anyway it gives one something to strive for!

Practice Technique

Lie down on your back and stretch out your arms behind your head (Fig. 29A). Feel the marvellous stretch from the tips of your fingers all the way down to your toes, and enjoy it for several seconds. Slowly start to raise your arms into a vertical position (Fig. 29B). Keeping your knees straight, sit up in one flowing movement, stretch, and inhale (Fig. 29C). Slowly bend forward while exhaling, and reach down as close to your feet as possible, ideally curling your index fingers around your big toes (working out the feet and ligaments of the legs as well). Totally motionless, hold this pose for ten seconds (Fig. 29D). Keeping your head way down, slowly come out of this posture, letting your hands slide over your legs and tightening your abdomen at the same time. When you return into a sitting position, clasp your hands together behind your back, raise them high, and lift your chin as in the Swan (Fig. 17A). Breathe in, hold for five seconds, exhale, and relax.

29C

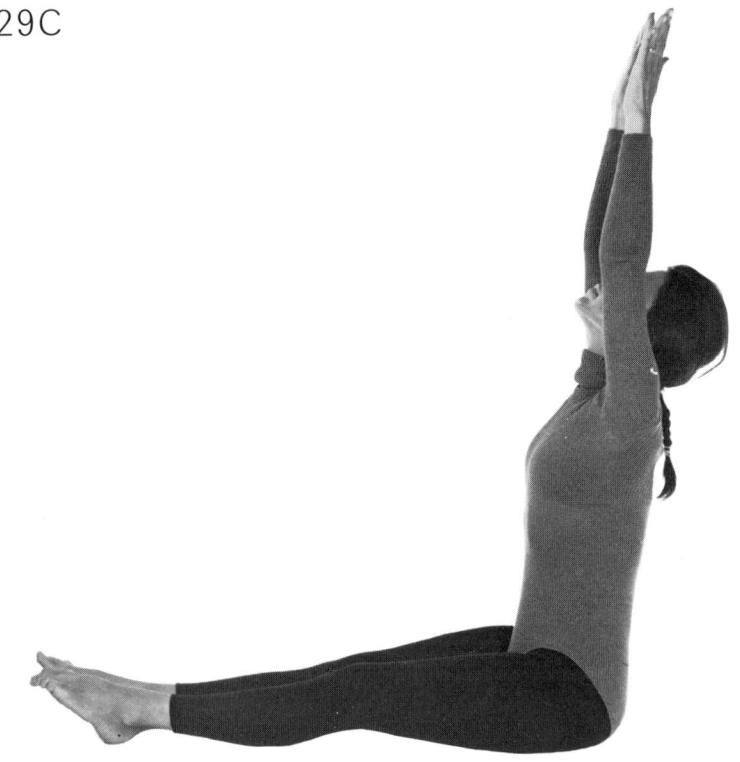

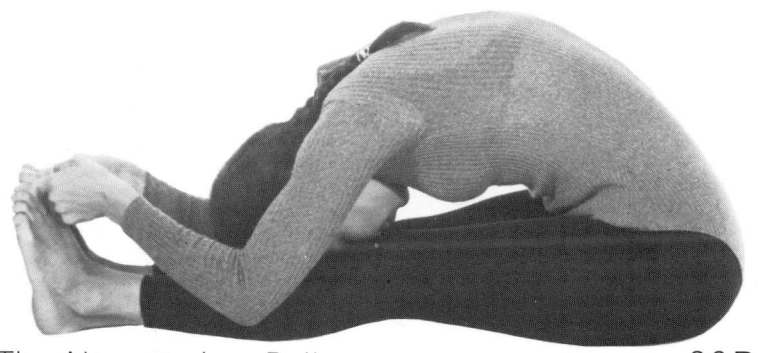

The Alternate Leg Pull   29D

Keep your knees and legs straight for this one, too.

Practice Technique

Sit on the floor, your left leg stretched straight out in front of
you, the right sole closely pressed toward the groin. Body
centred. Stretch your arms up high and breathe in (Fig. 30A).

30A

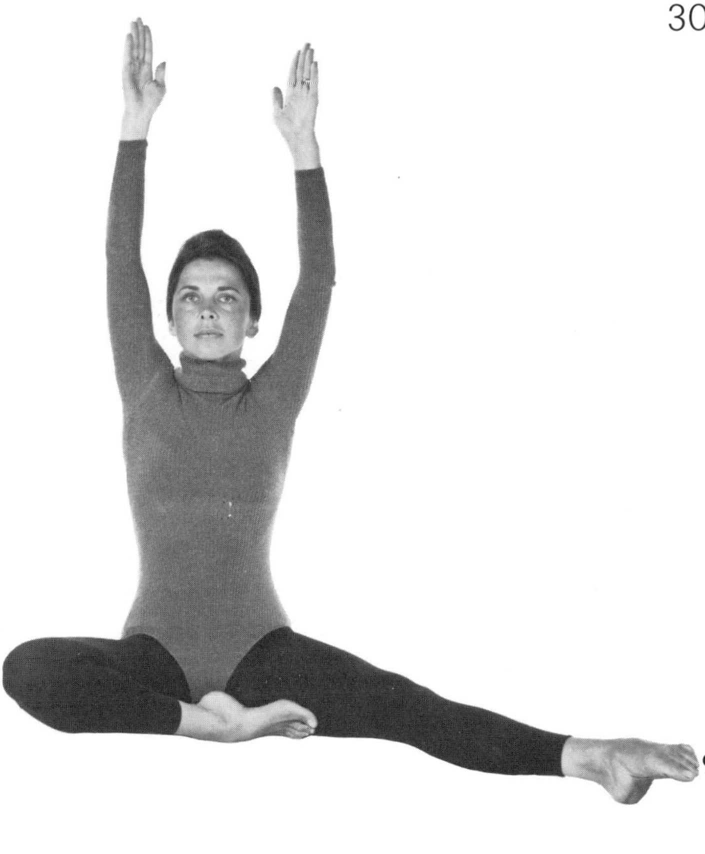

Slowly bend forward while inhaling, and reach down as far as you possibly can. Try to curl your index fingers around your big toe. If this is easy for you to do, bend the elbows to give an ultimate stretch to the body (Fig. 30B). Close your eyes, relax your neck and keep your head all the way down, holding this posture for ten seconds. Eventually work the time up to thirty-five seconds. Slowly come up, keeping your head way down, sliding your hands over your leg while tightening your abdomen as well. After you have returned to a sitting position, conclude this posture with the Swan pose by clasping your hands together behind your back, raising them way up high, chin held up, breathing in and holding for five seconds, exhaling, and then relaxing. Repeat on alternate side.

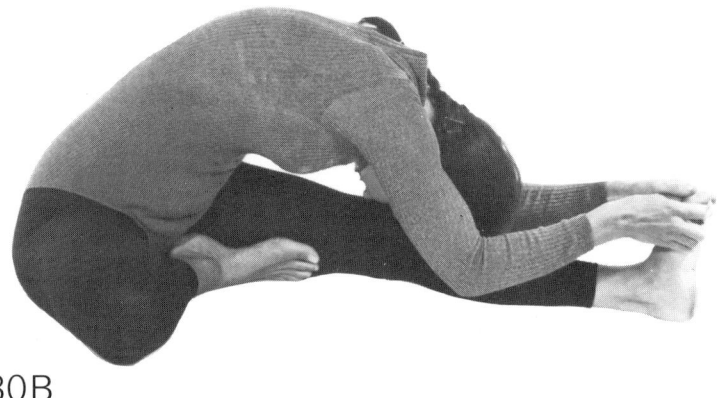

30B

The Ankle and Thigh Stretch
This is the only posture in this book that will and should hurt. But since it can't be harmful if you don't allow yourself to strain, console yourself with the thought that it is a terrific posture for tightening up those thigh muscles!

Practice Technique
Sit on the floor and place the soles of your feet against one another (Fig. 31A). Press your knees down and pull your feet in and up with both hands. Slowly bend your head as far forward as you can (Fig. 31B). Hold for ten seconds or as long as you can possibly stand it.

94

31A

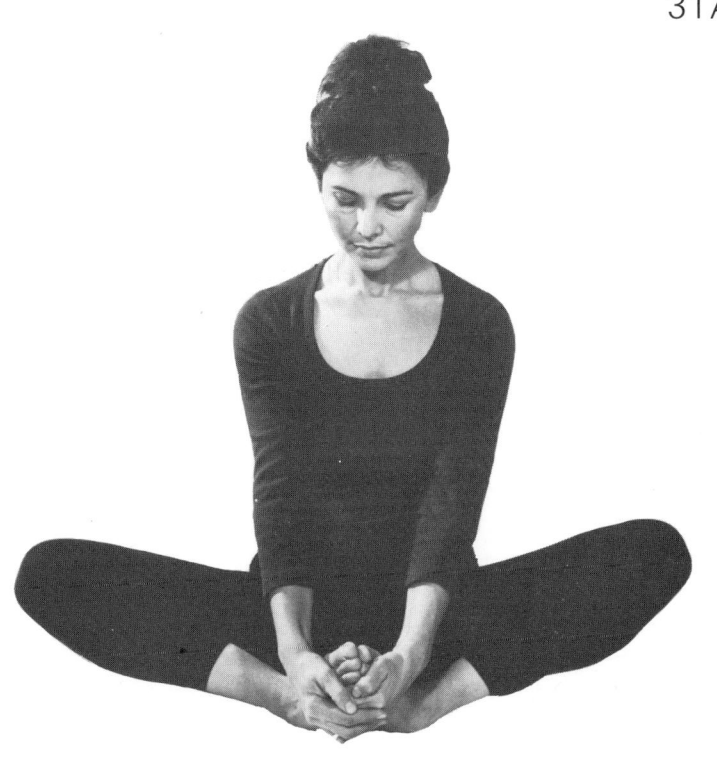

31B

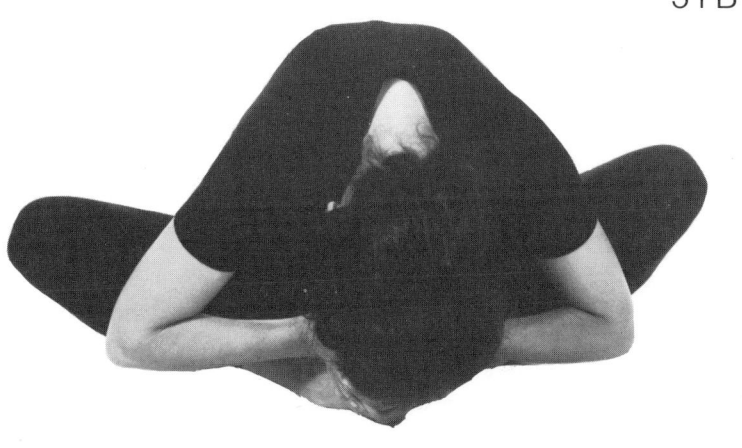

Chapter Thirteen

Anger, jealousy and greed are emotions that obscure the mind like heavy clouds that separate us from the sun. Let self-awareness become the wind whose force can drive away the curtain of darkness.

Deep Relaxation

Relaxation is actually more difficult than most of us think. In fact, many people don't know how to relax properly—after a day of rushing and running around, meeting deadlines, frustrations, and tension, many of us are too keyed up and tired to unwind, even while asleep. We toss and turn and our anxieties pursue us even in our dreams. The next morning we are almost as tired as before we went to sleep. And we do need good sleep very much for it is during our sleep that our body accumulates the energy needed for our daily work, activities, and emotions. Unfortunately, we have created our own monster. How often do we start the day in nerve-grinding traffic jams, making us long for a deserted island far away, or find ourselves packed like sardines on the tube, wondering whether the blasted thing is ever going to move on. By the time we get to our destination we are either late for work, have missed an important appointment, or maybe even that plane to India! Tension has built up, our nerves are rattled, and at the slightest frustration we explode, often at the people who mean the most to us.

It is not only physical strain and effort that uses up our energy. Anger, worry, and tension drain enormous amounts of energy from our body, leaving us tired and irritable. If we do not replenish this energy, the price we have to pay is great, for it ages our body and mind more rapidly. Therefore, the deep relaxation of Yoga is of great importance to our health. It revitalizes our body, regenerates the mind, and creates new life force to guide us with renewed strength, endurance, and patience throughout the remaining day.

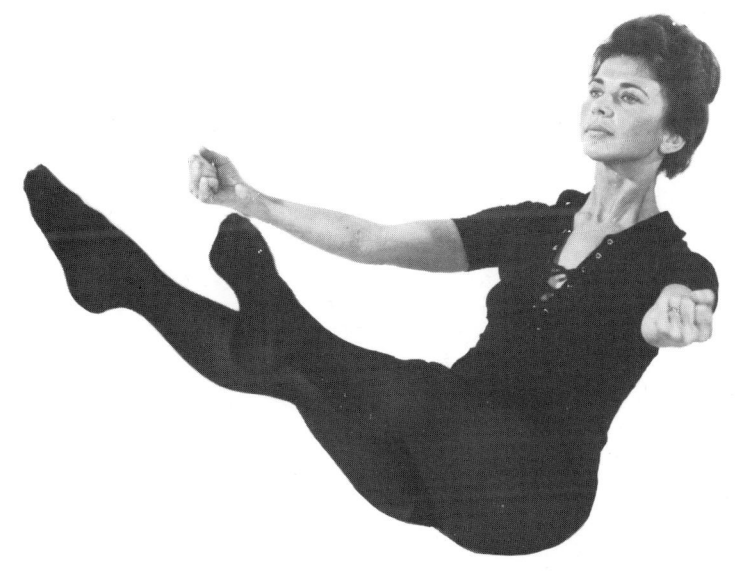

Savasana or Corpse Pose

Are you going out to the theatre tonight, or perhaps preparing a dinner party? Or are the children going to be home from school very soon? I know how busy you are, but do take ten or fifteen minutes out for the deep Yoga relaxation. It will reward you in so many ways. Tonight you will be a radiant and relaxed hostess, reaching out with warmth to your guests, making them feel good and completely at ease, the perfect ingredients for a lovely evening. What about sitting through that play and enjoying it, instead of dozing off in the middle! And when the children are home, you can listen to them with greater interest and better understanding. Isn't it worth a try?

Practice Technique
Disconnect that telephone for a while and lie down and relax for several seconds. All at once come up (Fig. 32A), vibrating every muscle in your body and limbs for ten slow seconds. Then let your body, arms, and legs drop heavily back to the floor and completely relax in the Corpse Pose (Fig. 32B). Close your eyes and concentrate on your feet and relax them.

Now relax your ankles, calves, knees, thighs. Tighten them for a moment and then relax them again. Your legs should feel heavy. Slowly work your way up, focusing your thoughts on each part of the body, making sure all muscles are loose and relaxed. The abdomen, buttocks, spine, and chest, all your muscles are slowly unwinding, the body is sinking deeper and deeper into a state of complete relaxation.

Check your shoulders, arms, hands, and fingers. Don't

32B

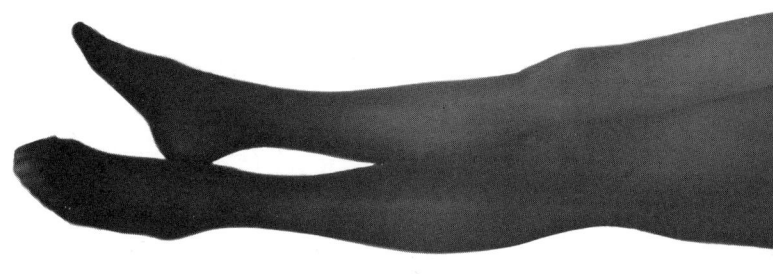

clench your hands. Relax. Concentrate on those muscles in
the neck where so much tension gathers, and slowly roll your
head to the right and to the left, to the right and to the left.
Let all thoughts wander from your mind. Breathe deeply and
slowly and allow your senses gently to melt into all that is
surrounding you. Enjoy the luxurious feeling of calmness and
tranquility.

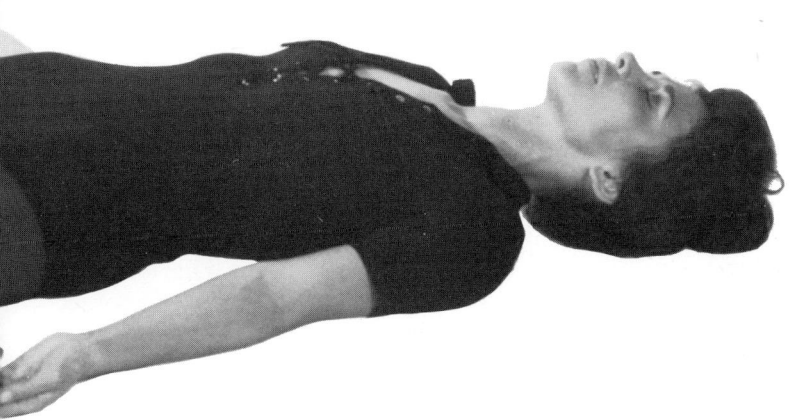

Chapter Fourteen

Yoga aims for a mind that is like the water of a spring, the clearness of which allows the light of the sun to reach the depth of its bottom.

Proper Breathing Through Yoga

Breathing is the very essence of life, yet it is hard to believe that so few of us correctly perform something that is as natural as breathing. Most of us breathe shallowly, using only the upper part of our lungs, neglecting, and therefore weakening, the abdominal or lower part of our lungs. The great Yoga masters claimed centuries ago, 'He who controls breath, controls life itself.' That sounds like something you might find in a Christmas cracker, but nevertheless there is a lot of truth to it. Today many leading physicians agree that correct breathing is of vital importance to our health. There is quite a variety of Yoga breathing that can help to achieve correct breathing, and I will proceed by discussing the three that are considered the most important.

The Complete Breath

The Complete Breath teaches us to use our lungs to their fullest capacity and to control the motions of our lungs. This technique will develop the breathing power of the lungs, which is of great importance to health and well-being. Not only will correct breathing affect one's physical condition but it will induce a state of mental and spiritual tranquillity. For the slow, deep flow of the breath will create a serenity and calmness of mind, just as the body will receive new energy and vitality by the great supply of life-giving oxygen that is led throughout the bloodstream. After practising Yoga breathing correctly and regularly, you should feel that your physical endurance has improved dramatically and find yourself to be out of breath far less soon during strenuous activities.

This breathing technique is often taught to actors and

singers, as it develops the ability to hold the breath much longer, therefore increasing the voice's volume and power of projection. It might even be of help when you are angry and upset. Nothing like taking a deep breath and holding it, giving you a few seconds to consider whether to go berserk or cool it! The Complete Breath is done in three stages: abdominal or deep breathing, chest or middle breathing, upper lung or high breathing. In this way the lungs are filled to their capacity with fresh air and a greater supply of energy can be sent through the body. The blood circulation is stimulated (which itself is excellent for the complexion) and more oxygen is fed to the brain. The total usage of the lungs also strengthens them, making them more elastic and increasing circulatory efficiency. Many people find that as a result they have greater resistance to colds and other respiratory ailments.

Practice Technique
The room should be well ventilated. Let the cool fresh air in, or, if you have a backyard or a garden, go outside on a lovely spring morning to practise the Yoga breathing. The effect will be exhilarating. You'll feel full of life and energy, your complexion will radiate and your eyes will become bright and clear.

Sit straight, using a cross-legged or, if you wish, a Half Lotus position. Exhale completely, relax your abdomen, and think of yourself as a deflated balloon (Fig. 33). Slowly extend your abdomen and begin to inhale gently. Without interrupting the inhalation, contract your abdomen and midriff, and, still inhaling, extend your chest. Then slowly raise your shoulders. Close your eyes and hold your breath for five seconds.

Yoga breathing emphasizes slow, long exhalation in order to empty the lungs of stale, stagnant air, and it is important to learn to control the exhalation so that it is as slow as possible. Ideally the exhalations should take twice as long as the inhalation, though it will require some time and practice to master this technique.

Repeat the Complete Breath three more times.

Note : This technique of inhalation and exhalation is done in one flowing motion. Some people might not be accustomed to the enormous amount of oxygen the body takes in during

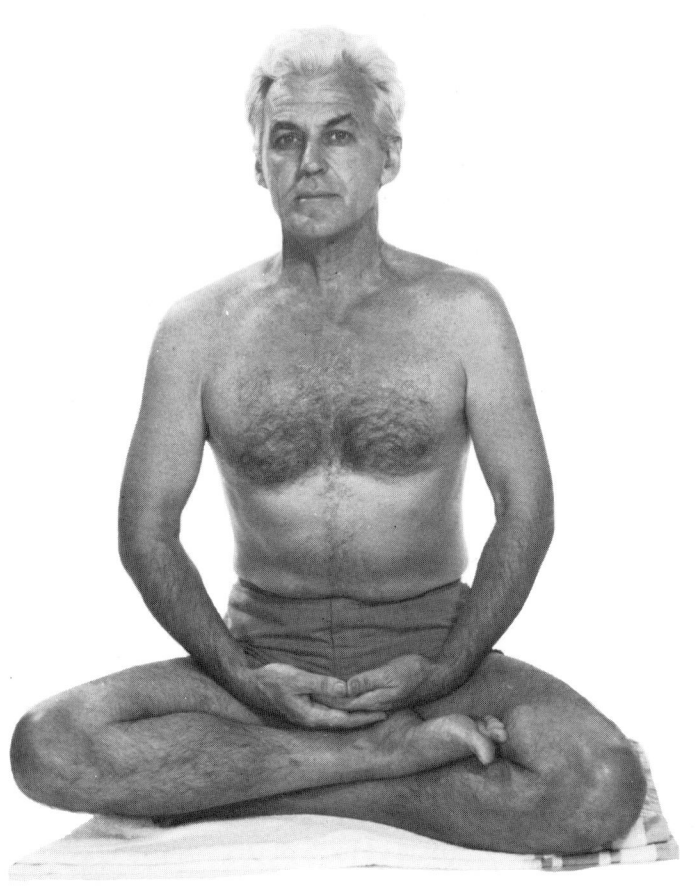

33

this exercise and could experience a slight light-headed
feeling. Therefore, time your breathing to your own ability.

The Abdominal Breath

This technique is called the Abdominal Breath because the
breathing is done from the abdomen and with the diaphragm.
It is sometimes called the Cleansing Breath as well since this
particular breathing technique cleanses the lungs and the
bronchia of carbon dioxide. It is accomplished by forceful
contractions of the abdominal muscles and the diaphragm,

which cause rapid, thrusting exhalations, thus forcing the stale air out of the periphery of the lung tissue. And the slow, long inhalations that follow fill the lungs with clean, oxygenated air and lead a greater supply of oxygen to the system, creating more alertness and a refreshing and vigorous sensation. After practising this particular breathing technique for a while, smokers will find that the inhaling of cigarette smoke becomes an irritant and an interference with the pure and clean feeling Yoga breathing has created in the lungs. I have found Yoga breathing was of tremendous help to me in 'kicking the smoking habit.' (I was also aided by the fact that for a year I feverishly knitted sweater after sweater, socks in all sizes, handfuls of mittens, and infinitely long scarfs, just to occupy my restless hands, meanwhile keeping my family wrapped in the result of my triumph!)

In the breathing process that is most commonly used, one contracts the abdomen while inhaling and extends while exhaling. The abdominal breathing is done in exactly the reversed way. Extended abdomen while inhaling, contracted abdomen while exhaling. Interestingly enough, we are born breathing this way but gradually change to the one mentioned previously. The abdominal breathing, however, is a far more healthy and effective way of breathing.

Practice Technique
Sit in a cross-legged or Half Lotus position, again making sure you are comfortable but straight. Relax your abdomen. To the count of three, slowly extend your abdomen while simultaneously inhaling (Fig. 34A). At the count of four, quickly snap the muscles in with force, which will compel you to exhale as well (Fig. 34B). Hold for a moment and repeat. Slowly inhale while extending the abdomen, exhale while contracting them forcefully, until you have completed ten expulsions. Continue for two more rounds, but rest between each round for several seconds by taking deep regular breaths. Every week you may add ten more expulsions to each round, until you have reached a total of fifty expulsions in each round.
Note : This is a rather strong breathing exercise which can be quite tiring if you are not used to it, and which can cause light-headedness because of the unaccustomed great intake

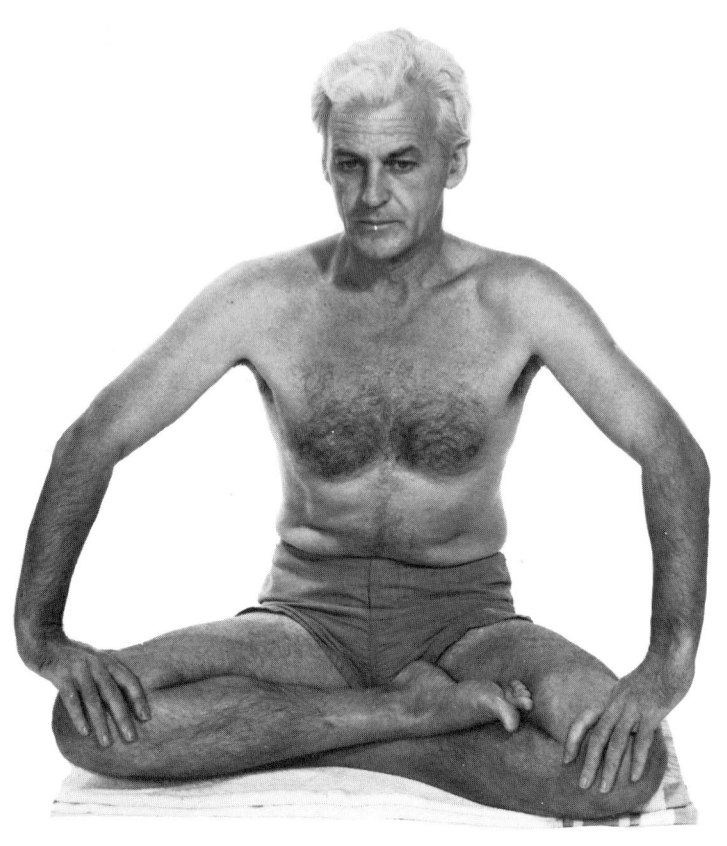

34A

of oxygen. It should be practised carefully and according to your own individual stamina. And since it is the reverse of our regular breathing, it will require some time, practice, and concentration to be mastered.

Alternate Nostril Breathing
This breathing technique has a most soothing and tranquilizing effect on the emotions. It calms the mind and is of great help to those who have difficulties falling asleep.

And for those who suffer from sinus problems or congestion, it will become a most important breathing exercise to practise

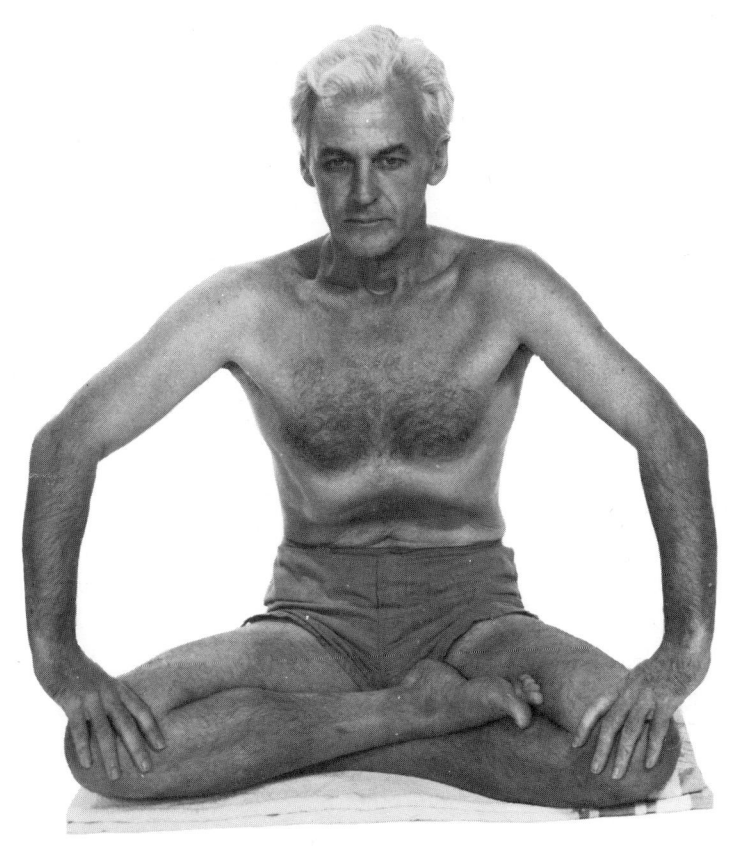

34B

since it will clear the sinuses remarkably well, making the breathing easier and more regular.

Practice Technique
Sit in cross-legged, Half Lotus (Full Lotus if you like) or in any erect but comfortable position.

Place the middle and index finger of your right hand on your forehead, just about between your eyebrows. Cover your right nostril with your thumb, and inhale deeply through your left nostril (Fig. 35). At the count of four, cover your left nostril with your ring and little fingers and hold your breath

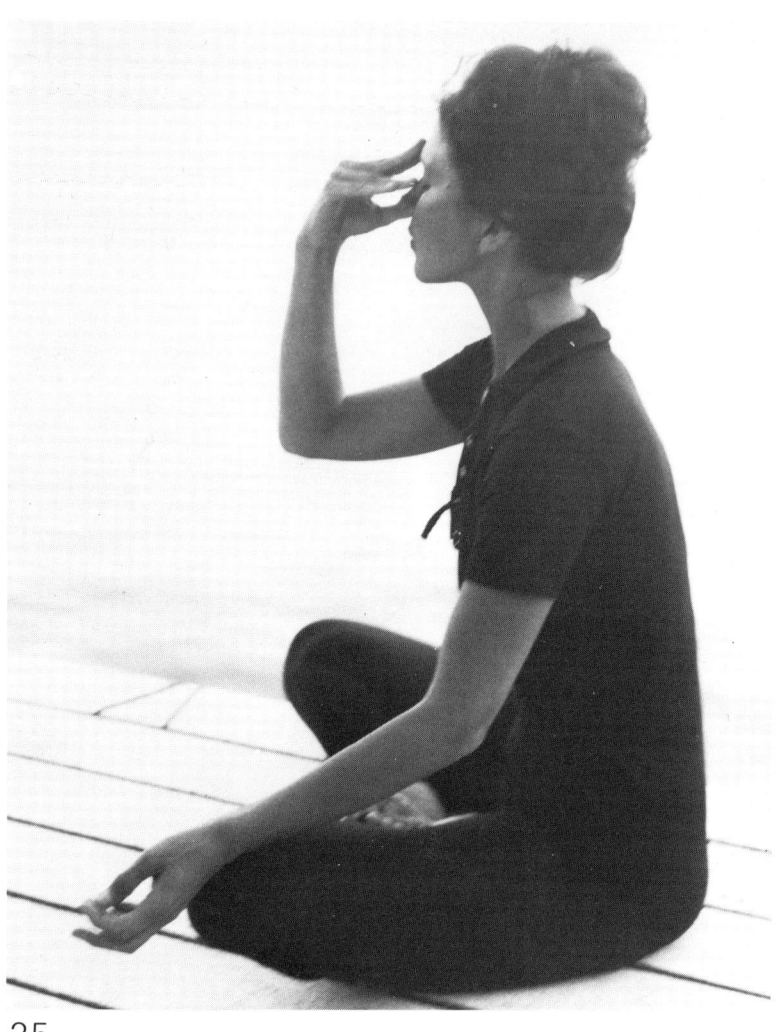

35

to the count of eight. Lift your thumb from your right nostril, and slowly exhale to the count of four. Without pausing, inhale through the right nostril to the count of four, cover the nostril with your thumb and hold your breath to the count of eight, lift the ring and little fingers from your left nostril and exhale. This is one full round, and should be done in one flowing motion. Continue for eight more rounds and slowly over a period of about two months work up to fifteen rounds.

But once again, use your judgment. Don't be in a hurry.

Chapter Fifteen

And when I touch
I will lead you through those heavy clouds
and help you reach the clear blue sky,
the sun so near it almost burns our bodies . . .
and when we plunge into the waves
we gently roll ashore, lying together closely,
not aware the sun went down, its penetrating warmth
glows deep inside us,
soft and long thereafter.

Yoga and Sex

When body and mind are as closely interrelated as in Yoga, we cannot ignore the important influence Yoga can have on our sexual lives. We can't live as whole human beings if our sexual drives and desires remain unfulfilled, for if these powerful forces that are throbbing within the human being are not gratifyingly released in a normal and healthy way, they not only can injure the body but distort the mind as well. Once we accept a wholesome sexual relationship as being as natural, functional, and enjoyable as eating and sleeping, we are on our way to beautiful and complete lives.

With Yoga, we can develop a heightened awareness of the sensitivity of the skin, muscles, and sexual organs that will enable us to increase all aspects of sexual pleasure and find a healthy delight in the pure sensations of our bodies.

Part of the total enjoyment begins when we are able to freely express our feelings and emotions without inhibitions or shame, and are liberated enough to explore the many varied ways one can experience pleasure: to touch, to laugh, and to be aware of oneself, but above all, to give joy and pleasure, for this will be returned in a most exciting and beautiful way.

Learn to relax your body and your mind, become aware of the sensitivity of your skin, the soft touch of fingers, listen to the heartbeat of the one you love, turn off the world around you and let the warm and lovely feelings take over body and soul. In this total harmony of two people, for one thrilling moment dissolving into one, you have discovered the true poetry of sex.

How does Yoga fit into one's sex life?

The new flexibility and awareness of our bodies allow a

greater freedom of movement, and as we learn to relax more deeply and to let go of physical strain and tension, our bodies will react more instinctively and naturally to their needs and become lovely instruments that enable us to find great joy in the wonderful simplicity of sexual delight. After all, doesn't the Kama Sutra claim 64 different positions possible in man's sex life, which does make things rather adventurous. Therefore isn't it great to feel limber, desirable, and sensuous!

Do take good care of your body, for it is an instrument that enables you to give and receive one of the greatest pleasures nature has given to man.

Keep it healthy, make it move graciously, and let it smell fresh. I don't mean for you to use a combination of cologne and deodorant, for there is nothing more delicious and earthy than the natural smell of a clean and healthy body. And some women are unaware that a minimum of makeup actually makes them look much softer and younger. Other than the chain and leather set, I doubt that there are many men who prefer to make love to a woman whose eyes are covered with mascara and false eyelashes (he might even swallow one), or to kiss thick lipstick, or to try to caress a head full of hair curlers. Nothing is more attractive than a soft natural hairstyle. When you need to set your hair, by all means do so in private, don't make love in it. This I have always considered an insult to oneself (not to mention to the other half—for some curlers look and feel like lethal weapons) and one of women's greatest sins!!

There is a mystique surrounding Yoga and its effect on sexual impulses. Sometimes I am asked in jest what this precisely entails, as if there must be some sordid answer to it. It is true though that women possess pelvic muscles that are often dormant and neglected, which is a pity, for the movements of these muscles can give tremendous stimulation and heighten pleasure to her and her partner. By relaxing and contracting these muscles thirty to thirty-five times a day as an exercise, one can make them extremely strong and flexible. (I've been told that in California there are waitresses so expert in this art that they can pick up a silver dollar—which can be most useful if one happens to have ones hands full!) Anyway, laugh, be happy, and enjoy. So few pleasures in life come free, make the most of this one.

108

Chapter Sixteen

Intelligence itself is not the measure of man, nor is only the yielding to emotions—but united they can form the balance of a wise and complete person.

Improving the Complexion Through Yoga

Millions of pounds are spent annually on cosmetics by men and women alike in the hope of attaining a healthy and flawless complexion. But I do believe that a beautiful complexion is more than skin deep, for this desirable image cannot be acquired out of bottles and jars. It involves a healthy, wholesome way of life. So let us first discuss some of the factors that can be so destructive to the complexion and then continue with constructive advice that can be of help to you in achieving a clear, natural lustre.

Most of us now live in centrally-heated houses. Not only are our bedrooms heated, but the bathrooms too, which is very comfortable. (I can still remember those days during my childhood in Holland when I used to wake up with frost on my blankets. The hardest thing to do was to get out of bed—though it did teach me to dress fast.) In the Northern European countries, however, where the climate is cool and damp, bedrooms are often not centrally heated and you find that the people have a beautiful, healthy complexion. After all, central heating dries out furniture, is devastating for a piano, and unhealthy for plants, so it stands to reason that it will dry out your skin as well. I have the heat turned off in all the bedrooms, and sleep with open windows (one has to ignore the soot of large cities). But if you find it difficult to sleep in such a cool bedroom, by all means invest in a good humidifier.

Most public buildings, such as schools, office buildings and department stores are also overheated, and it would be much healthier for the people in them (and more economical for whoever is footing the bill) if temperatures were kept lower. Besides the heat drying out the skin, it makes people tired and drowsy and lessens their resistance to the cold temperatures outside.

Another thing that can make the skin look drawn and grey is lack of sleep. We do require a certain amount of sleep, and if we are tired it shows in our face and our eyes become strained and dull. One should really allow oneself at least eight hours of sleep. Of course, there are times when, for many different reasons, we don't get the right amount of sleep. In this case, try to make up for it during the day. If you learn the art of deep Yoga relaxation (Chapter 13), you will find that it enables you completely to rest the body and the mind within a short span of time, producing a regenerating effect that provides the stamina needed to move effectively and productively throughout the day. Sleep and relaxation are not luxuries. They are essential for your well-being!

Alcohol is another enemy of the complexion. Of course, this does not mean an occasional cocktail or a glass of wine with dinner, but regular or excessive drinking. Alcohol goes into our bloodstream and eventually enlarges the capillaries, creating a red and bloated complexion. And while we are at it, cigarettes are not good for us either. I'm sure you have heard that before, but since we have such a hard time finding pure, clean air to breathe, why add insult to injury? Smoking does affect the respiratory system and limits the amount of life-giving oxygen that enters our bloodstream. I was once told by a very concerned friend that with every cigarette I smoked I aged. That was probably a slight exaggeration, but it was all I had to hear to get me started on my 'knitting madness' and doing the Yoga breathing exercises described in Chapter 14.

Finally, let us discuss one of the greatest of all evils for the skin, the sun. And I happen to be a sunworshipper, spending endless summer hours on the beach. But, alas, as we grow older, our skin becomes drier. This is an inevitable, natural process and all we can do about it is to avoid the situations that can accelerate it. Now, you don't have to sit under a parasol or stroll the beaches clad in yards of veil, but do avoid overexposure. Time your sunbathing carefully. I have found that for me a daily sunbath of half an hour, preferably around eleven o'clock or four o'clock when the sun is not so strong, will create a soft glowing, golden tan. But at all times grease yourself!! Use anything that is oily, such as suntan lotion,

Vaseline, or baby oil. But whichever you choose never sun-bathe without it or you will end up with a complexion that resembles an elephant hide!

And now that we know what is bad for us, let's find out what is good for us.

The golden rule: Always keep the skin clean. I like soap and water provided it is a rich emollient soap. But I'm aware that many people consider soap skin's worst enemy, so for them there is an assortment of astringent lotions which clean effectively and refresh the skin at the same time.

I also consider vitamin E an important aid and skin treatment. After thirty, the body slows down its production of natural oils, and as we grow older it becomes of vital importance to supplement this deficiency. This can be done quite successfully by a regular, daily intake of vitamin E. At the same time, one should use vitamin E externally as well. By simply punching a hole in the capsule with a pin and spreading the oil over the face, it will serve as a rich and most nourishing overnight treatment for the skin.

Another marvellous skin treatment is the old-fashioned mask made out of egg whites. (In case you like your egg white flavoured, add several drops of lemon juice). Let the whites harden on the face—it looks and feels ghastly, but the effect is gorgeous. Afterward, rinse with cool water.

And don't cover your face with too much makeup, for the skin has to breathe. But whether you are wearing makeup or not, always use a moisturizer during the day. I would try to avoid powder, for it creates a dull effect and dries out the skin. It really doesn't matter if the face shines a little—in fact it will be more natural and healthy looking.

Since our physical condition plays an important role in the way we look, walk a lot. It is healthy for the body and also good for the complexion. Don't let the rain or cold weather stop you, just bundle up and breathe deeply.

In addition to the deep breathing exercises, Yoga postures such as Shoulderstand (Fig. 4A) and the Headstand (Fig. 5D) bring a lovely colour and a healthy lustre to the face. At the same time, these postures stimulate the scalp and therefore nourish the hair roots, giving sheen to dull, lifeless hair and controlling loss of hair.

I realize this has turned into a rather austere chapter. No

smoking, or drinking, early to bed, and as if this is not bad enough, sleeping in what may seem to you subzero temperatures. But at least I let you breathe and enjoy your sex life!

Here are two Yoga exercises that will help bring sparkle to your eyes and firmness to your face:

Eye Exercise

Our eyes reflect the way we feel, and in them lies the evidence of a tense and tiring day. We can relieve tension and remove fatigue with this marvellous eye-exercise that acts as a refreshing tonic while, in addition, it strengthens the optic nerves and exercises the eye muscles.

Practice Technique
Keep your head absolutely motionless. Pretend your eyes are following the hands of a clock. Look all the way up, starting at twelve, go clockwise to three, six, nine, and back to twelve. Repeat this four times. Then do it counterclockwise, four times.

Now rub your palms together, to create heat. Gently place the palms over your eyes, and let the eyes absorb the warmth and darkness for a while. When your eyes are rested, remove your hands.

The Lion

Just as Yoga postures firm and tighten the muscles in our body, they can do the same for the face.

The weakening and therefore sagging of the facial muscles will be counteracted dramatically by the consistent practice of the Lion, whose profound muscular movement delays and reduces wrinkles and crows' feet, and stretches away strain and tension lines.

The simple movement of this exercise works out the most essential muscles in our face and has the great advantage that it can be performed any time, at any place, though it seems I have just scared away the photographer!

Practice Technique
Make big eyes and roll them all the way up. Now stick your tongue out as far as possible (Fig. 36) and hold this position for fifteen seconds. Relax and repeat four times.

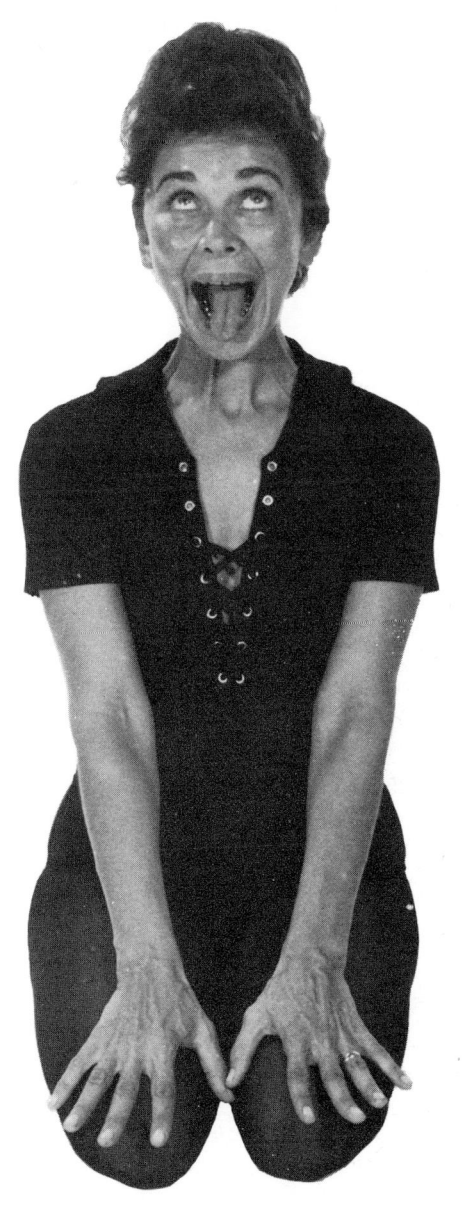

Chapter Seventeen

Let us remember that inside each of us is someone who at times feels lonely and afraid, insecure and unloved, secretly hoping that another will have the strength to reach out beyond the defensive wall that surrounds us.

The Power of Control Over Body and Mind

For centuries Western philosophers and psychologists have speculated about the relationship between the body and the mind. Until early in this century, the more 'modern' scientists attempted to dismiss the entire question by considering it an artificial, semantic problem.

At the same time, however, it was becoming evident both in the West and the East, that there is in fact a real connection between mind and body and that this connection could be demonstrated. In the West, increasing evidence indicated that a wide range of physical illnesses and disabilities could be caused by the mind. These diseases included peptic ulcers, asthma, colitis, and migraine headaches.

More and more people with these illnesses were referred to psychiatrists whose treatment of the mind repaired the disorders of the body.

Meanwhile, reports were coming in from scientists and visitors to India, describing a variety of phenomena observed in Yogis who through many years of Yoga learning and practice could influence and control the functioning of various body organs which theretofore had not been considered amenable to conscious control. Among these phenomena were the slowing of the heartbeat and increased resistance to pain shown by the classic performance of sleeping on a bed of nails. (It is interesting to note that the Indian word for someone who can swallow glass or lie on a bed of nails is fakir, and the English word faker is derived from the disbelief of early Western observers that this could actually be possible.)

Western scientists are now very interested in this relation between body and mind. Medical experiments have recently described how patients who are suffering from migraine headaches are taught, by conscious control of the internal processes causing these headaches, to alter the size of their blood vessels, thus relieving the throbbing pain, and in many cases, with significant improvement of the ailment. This technique represented one of the first practical applications of the human mind's ability to control internal organs—an ability that Westerners have seldom used intentionally and that many doubted possible. This will be a most interesting and fruitful field of discovery in future years.

This treatment employs a principle that Yogis have known for centuries, that many of the body's internal organs that seem to function and malfunction automatically, can be regulated by one's will. Many of the Yoga postures, as well as the deep relaxation and breathing techniques, are the preliminary steps along the path of gaining a healthy balance between the body and the mind.

So, in this sense, much of what I have tried to teach you through this book can become a form of preventive medicine.

Although this book concerns itself with the physical aspect of Yoga (Hatha Yoga), I would like to include a few words here about meditation (Raja Yoga), for it is a vital part of the beauty and strength of Yoga.

Let me try to give you a simplified explanation of the phenomenon of meditation.

When a baby is born it comprehends no difference or limitation between itself and the world. Its existence is simply a prolongation of the womb. This is a beautiful, blissful, as well as painless state to be in, with relatively few anxieties, fears, or frustrations. As the infant develops and matures, it begins to differentiate between itself and the world around it. This growing awareness forms the basis and nucleus of the developing personality, and it is also the beginning of the long process of growing up, with all its forces of joy, beauty, and passion, as well as pain, frustration, and anxiety.

As schizophrenic illness represents an unsuccessful attempt to return to an early blissful state, meditation is a *positive* attempt to recapture, for a limited period of time, this state of total oneness between oneself and the world, producing the feeling of peace, harmony, and unity with the universe that one was able to experience as an infant.

That is, in short, how meditation creates a restoring, revitalizing, and regenerating state of mind, which enables us once again to emerge and deal more effectively and harmoniously with the daily problems of life.

Although the method practice of meditation has been written in many books, I do not feel qualified to do so. Nor can this most interesting but delicate technique of deep meditation easily be conveyed in writing. Instead, I advise that if you are interested in the practice of deep meditation, you seek out a trained and experienced master of meditation and be taught under his personal guidance and instruction.

Chapter Eighteen

Every one of us is an individual with his own potential and limitations. Therefore, in Yoga we compete only with ourselves, each of us trying to reach the ultimate of our possibilities.

What Is It All About?

There comes a moment in everyone's life when he must ask himself, What is the meaning of life, why am I here, what is it all about? A universal and everlasting quest on which throughout the centuries volumes have been written by great and wise philosophers, poets, playwrights, and novelists, each in his own way trying to suggest the answer to the purpose of our existence and to find the reason for our being. But we continue to search, hoping to find the answer to it ourselves, for only then will we be able to truly understand.

Certainly I don't consider myself intelligent or wise enough to even attempt to answer a question of such immense depth, but perhaps I may tell you how I look at life and how I try to deal with it in my own way. I see life as an empty canvas given to us on the day we are born. The control we develop over our body and mind will serve as the tools we paint with; the growing of our awareness, senses, and emotions will be the colours of our paint; our deeds and actions will become the context and meaning we will give to our painting.

While we hesitantly put down those first lines to give shape to what we are trying to express, we gradually learn, often by trial and error, how we can give depth and dimension, shading and stronger feelings to what we are doing. We realize that each stroke has a meaning and an importance of its own. We experience that certain colours can create a radiant brilliance or can melt into a soft and tender composition. Compassion, honesty, and love are beautifully strong, bright colours to work with and serve perfectly as primary colours to blend with and mellow the darker and more dreary ones.

While the painting develops character, takes form and deeper meaning, some realize there must be many more ways to improve oneself and to learn more, and so we go out into the world to search for a better technique, to develop a style of our own or to expose ourselves to new experiences that will help to make us grow as artists in the hope of creating a painting that will express the richness of our emotions and the depth of our soul.

There will be moments when we become tired of our painting, or unhappy with the way it is turning out, doubtful of what we are doing. But it is not too late to correct what went wrong, to try to brighten the dullness of the colours or even to begin a different theme. Some of our work will turn out to be romantic, some realistic, others primitive, and a few of us will succeed in creating a true masterpiece.

Naturally all of us long for admiration and recognition. We do want people to like and understand what we are painting. But most rewarding and meaningful is that moment when you stand back to evaluate your own work and you can say, 'It is all right. I like what I have done.'

Afterword

By exercising, breathing, and relaxing, we have created a strength and energy in ourselves, increased and stimulated the respiratory system, and limbered and strengthened our bodies. And with this newly released energy, we have developed a power and vitality within ourselves which enables us to feed these forces back again into our environment, causing an electrifying effect around us, making us feel happy, healthy, and alive.

With this book I hope to have helped you gain health, youthfulness, and perhaps some fleeting moments of happiness. Youth, by helping you to develop a trim, limber, and graceful body and an awareness of the powers that are in all of us; health, through proper breathing, exercising, and the beautiful art of relaxation; happiness by making you smile, for if we cannot laugh at ourselves and the world around us any longer, we might as well stop breathing.

Do remember sometimes that we have been given the most powerful and unique instrument on earth, the human body. That we have legs that can take us to the top of the mountain, hands that touch, ears that hear, and eyes that see the sunlight.

Please, breathe deeply, hold, and exhale slowly!

Daily Practice Tables

Practice Table for the Beginner

Sit in comfortable Lotus position: *19*
The Complete Breath *P 100*
The Abdominal Contraction *P 79*
The Waistroll *P ~~76~~ 76*
The Alternate Leg Pull *P 93*
The Ankle and Thigh Stretch *P 94*
The Swan *P 67-79*
The Cat *P 48*
The Half Spinal Twist *P 44*
The Neck Stretch *P 65*
The Vibration Posture *P 75*
The Lion *P 112*
The Eye Exercise *P 112*

Stand up:
Salutation to the Sun *P 16*
Rishi's Posture *P 55*
The Dancer's Posture (First Stage) *P 59*
The Triangle *P 76*
The Chest Expansion (First Stage) *P 70*
The Corpse Pose *P 97*

Lie down on the back:
The Shoulderstand (First Stage) *P 26*
The Fish (First Stage) *P 481*
The Plow (First Stage) *P 40*

Turn over on the stomach:
The Half Locust *P 8 7*
The Cobra *p 3 6*

Turn over on the back: *P*
The Boat *P 8 1*
The Leg Pull *P9 1*
The Alternate Nostril Breathing *P 104*

Intermediate Practice Table

Sit in your comfortable Lotus position:
The Complete Breath *P 100*
The Cleansing Breath
The Waistroll *P 76*
The Alternate Leg Pull *P 9 3*
The Ankle and Thigh Stretch *P 9 4*
The Ultimate Body Stretch
The Yoga Seal
The Half Spinal Twist
The Warrior
The Neck Stretch
The Vibration Posture
The Lion
The Eye Exercise
The Monkey Posture

Stand up:
Salutation to the Sun
The Tree
The Full Dancer's Posture
The Triangle
The Chest Expansion (First and Second Stage)
The Head-to-Knee Pose
The Corpse Pose

Lie down on the back:
The Shoulderstand (Second Stage)
The Fish (Second Stage)
The Plow (First and Second Stage)
The Pelvic Stretch

122

Turn over on the stomach:
The Half and Full Locust
The Cobra

Turn over on the back:
The Boat
The Leg Pull
The Abdominal Contraction
The Alternate Nostril Breathing

The Advanced Practice Table

Sit in your most comfortable Lotus position:
The Complete Breath
The Cleansing Breath
The Waistroll
The Swan
The Alternate Leg Pull
The Upward Leg Pull
The Ankle and Thigh Stretch
The Camel and Child's Poses
The Yoga Seal
The Ultimate Body Stretch
The Cat
The Full Spinal Twist
The Warrior
The Neck Stretch
The Vibration Posture
The Lion
The Eye Exercise
The Monkey Posture

Come up in standing position:
Salutation to the Sun
Rishi's Posture
The Dancer's Posture (First and Second Stage)
The Tree
The Triangle
The Chest Expansion
The Head-to-Knee Pose
The Corpse Pose

Lie down on the back:
The Advanced Shoulderstand
The Fish
The Headstand
The Plow (First, Second, and Third Positions)
The Pelvic Stretch

Turn over on the stomach:
The Half Locust
The Full Locust
The Cobra

Return on the back:
The Boat
The Leg Pull
The Abdominal Contraction
The Alternate Nostril Breathing

Filmset in Monophoto Imprint by
Trade Spools, Frome, Somerset and
printed and bound in Great Britain by
Tinling (1973) Ltd. Prescot, Lancs.